80-00

MANIPULATION AND MOBILIZATION
EXTREMITY AND SPINAL TECHNIQUES

80-00

Manipulation and Mobilization Extremity and Spinal Techniques

SUSAN L. EDMOND, M.P.H., P.T.
Graduate Program in Physical Therapy
Simmons College
Boston, Massachusetts

LEE SHIONIS
Photography

CHERYL HARRINGTON
Illustrations

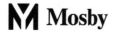 **Mosby**

St. Louis Baltimore Boston Chicago London Philadelphia Sydney Toronto

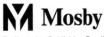 **Mosby**

Dedicated to Publishing Excellence

Sponsoring Editor: David Marshall
Assistant Editor: Julie Tryboski
Assistant Managing Editor, Text and Reference: George Mary Gardner
Production Supervisor: Carol A. Reynolds
Proofroom Manager: Barbara M. Kelly

1 2 3 4 5 6 7 8 9 0   CL MA   97 96 95 94 93

Library of Congress Cataloging-in-Publication Data
Edmond Susan L.
    Manipulation and mobilization : extremity and spinal techniques /
Susan L. Edmond.
      p. cm.
    Includes bibliographical references and index.
    ISBN 0-8016-6305-9
    1. Manipulation (Therapeutics)   2. Extremities (Anatomy)—
Diseases—Physical therapy.   3. Spine—Diseases—Physical therapy.
I. Title.
    [DNLM: 1. Manipulation, Orthopedic—methods.   WB 535 E24m]
RD736.M25E35   1992
615.8′ 2—dc20   92-49998
DNLM/DLC   CIP
for Library of Congress

PREFACE

Over the past decade, medical care has grown by leaps and bounds in terms of the technical complexity and sophistication of techniques directed at diagnosing and treating medical illnesses. Because of these technical advancements, the medical profession has grown increasingly reliant on tests and procedures utilizing complex instrumentation. One result of this advancement in medical technology is that diagnosing and healing by the laying on of hands is becoming increasingly rare. Thus in medical care, as it is practiced today, patient-clinician interaction often is minimal.

Manual therapy as practiced in the evaluation and treatment of orthopedic conditions is one of the few areas of medical care that rely on patient-clinician interaction, both verbally and by hands-on management. As such, it has evolved into both an art and a science. As a graduating physical therapist, I was fascinated by the power of manual techniques, and strived to master them. When I began teaching it was the subject matter I naturally gravitated to.

This book was conceived as a manual for use with entry-level physical therapy students as an aid in laboratory sessions. Because I believe a graduate education should promote in students an ability to self-learn, this book was designed to allow students to teach themselves manual techniques with minimal direction and demonstration from course instructors. I feel strongly that students and therapists thus empowered are capable of more independent and creative patient care. This book is thus designed as a self-learning tool for students and clinicians who seek to advance their understanding of evaluation and treatment techniques involving manipulation and mobilization of the extremities and spine, as part of their development as manual therapists.

Susan L. Edmond, M.P.H., P.T.

ACKNOWLEDGMENTS _____

Joann Brooks, whose advice and support while writing this book were invaluable, and who contributed her time to pose for photographs reproduced in this book.

Nora Robbins, whose artistic and design expertise added much to the quality of the photographs in this book.

Simmons College Media Center for their time and patience and use of their equipment while preparing photographs.

My students and colleagues for their inspiration and insight.

The staff at Mosby for their expertise in the editing and composition of this book.

Susan L. Edmond, M.P.H., P.T.

CONTENTS

Chapter 1

Introduction

Manipulation is defined in the *New Standard Dictionary of the English Language* as an "examination or treatment by the hands."[1] Whereas some practitioners more narrowly define joint manipulation as a specific technique in which the articular capsule is stretched by delivering a quick thrust maneuver to the joint, this definition provides ample argument for using the term joint manipulation to include any manual technique applied to a joint in dysfunction that moves the two surfaces in relation to one another. Included in this definition is joint manipulation in the more narrow sense; joint mobilization, which is a slow, passive movement imparted to an articular surface; and muscle energy, which is a technique in which the joint is moved by active contraction of the patient's muscle. Joint manipulation therefore can be defined as a manual therapeutic technique involving movement of one articular surface in relation to another that is performed on an articular structure that has been shown to be in dysfunction on physical examination.

Joint manipulation has been a part of medicine since recorded history. There is evidence of manual techniques being used in Thailand in 2000 B.C. as well as in ancient Egypt. Hippocrates used manual traction in the treatment of spinal deformities. In the United States and Europe during the more recent 1800s, practitioners referred to as bonesetters developed an entire practice consisting of joint manipulation techniques.[2] Although they were ignorant of much of the anatomic and physiologic bases for manipulation, these practitioners used a series of techniques that were often successful in reducing pain and deformity.

Chiropractic and osteopathic medicine originated in the early 20th century. Many of the techniques practiced by chiropractors and osteopaths resembled those of the bonesetters. Both chiropractic and osteopathic medicine are based on the premise that disease, including spinal disorders, is due to vertebral dysfunction. Chiropractors emphasized the role of the spinal nerve in the cause of disease, and osteopaths emphasized the role of the vertebral arteries. Many chiropractors now recognize that most diseases cannot be cured by spinal manipulations, and they limit their treatments to spinal dysfunction. Osteopaths continue to use manipulation as an adjunct to treatment, but have expanded their training to include that of medical physicians. In the United States, osteopaths currently have the same training as medical physicians, with the additional training in manipulation. Much of our current knowledge of manipulative therapy comes from osteopathy.

While few clinicians currently believe that there is a direct relationship between spinal dysfunction and disease, there is still some acknowledgment of the role of vertebral dysfunction in the cause of nonvertebral disorders. Many practitioners recognize that when an element of the skeletal, arthrodial, or myofascial system is in dysfunction, alterations in related vascular, lymphatic, and neural systems occur.[2] The specifics of the connection between manipulation and systemic dysfunction have not been clearly outlined; however, examples of its existence are apparent in clinical practice. For instance, complaints by patients of dizziness after even gentle upper cervical manipulations are not uncommon and are considered to be related to systemic neurologic alterations due to the manipulation techniques.

Other practitioners who have contributed to the knowledge base of manipulative therapy include James Cyriax, John M. Mennell, Robert Maigne, G.D. Maitland, and Freddy Kaltenborn. Cyriax was an orthopedic physician who contributed much to the development of a system of physical examination in which the different tissues affected by orthopedic disorders are selectively isolated and tested. He also brought into common usage some of the manipulative techniques practiced today, particularly those used for the treatment of spinal disc disorders. Mennell developed the concept that adhesions are a common cause of joint dysfunction. Maigne believed that a clinician should not perform a treatment that increases the patient's symptoms, and therefore treatment should be administered in a direction opposite the direction that reproduces pain. Maitland developed oscillatory manipulation treatments and stated, in contradiction to Maigne, that one should oscillate in the direction of reproducible symptoms. Kaltenborn proposed that the clinician should treat with oscillations in a direction based on analysis of the restriction in range of motion and the articular surface anatomy. Also worthy of mention for their roles in the development of manipulative therapy are Stanley Paris and Ola Grimsby, who did much to disseminate information regarding manipulation to clinicians. Paris proposed that the clinician should treat joint dysfunction and minimize the role of pain. In this book, an attempt is made to draw on and consolidate the different philosophies and to present a system of treatment of joint manipulation as is commonly practiced by physical therapists.

INDICATIONS

All joints are capable of physiologic movement. Physiologic movement occurs when muscles contract concentrically or eccentrically or when gravity acts on a bone to move it. This type of movement is classified as osteokinematic motion. The different directions of motion of which each joint is capable is called its osteokinematic degrees of freedom. A maximum of six different degrees of freedom are possible in each joint: four degrees of freedom occur as the bone moves in either direction in two planes of motion perpendicular to one another, and two occur as the bone rotates around an axis perpendicular to the joint surfaces.

Joints also undergo arthrokinematic movement, which is motion between two articulating surfaces without reference to the forces being applied to that joint. Arthrokinematic motion in each joint also is characterized by a specific number of degrees of freedom. This is determined by the amount of accessory motion present in a particular articulation. Accessory motion, or joint play, is joint motion that is not under voluntary control, yet is necessary for pain-free, unrestricted voluntary movement to occur. Joint manipulation entails moving a joint through its accessory motion.

The goal of manipulation is to restore maximal, pain-free movement to a musculoskeletal system, which is in postural balance.[2] Joint manipulation accomplishes this goal in the following ways.

Increasing Joint Extensibility

Joint manipulation promotes optimal, pain-free movement by maintaining extensibility of joint and other periarticular structures or by increasing extensibility in the presence of periarticular restrictions. Restrictions in the joint capsule usually are accompanied by a corresponding limitation in joint range of motion.

Restrictions are usually the result of either immobilization or inflammation of articular and surrounding structures. When the joint is immobilized, a number of changes occur in the joint capsule. Intracellular water content decreases, resulting in a decrease in the distance between fibers constituting the joint capsule. This results in an increase in fiber cross-link formation, which produces adhesions. Immobilization also produces adhesions between synovial folds. During the immobilization, new collagen tissue is produced, and if movement does not occur between these tissues, additional cross-linking will occur. Immobilization also produces fibrofatty connective tissue proliferation within the joint, which is transformed into scar tissue. In addition, the strength of collagen tissue decreases, resulting in a decrease in the load-to-failure rate.

Joint manipulation is thought to reverse these changes by promoting movement between capsular fibers. This is believed to result in an increase in interstitial water content and inter-fiber distance. It also is believed that by promoting movement between capsular fibers through the repetitive manipulation of joint structures, synovial tissue will stretch in a selective manner, causing a gradual rearrangement of old collagen tissue with a reduction of cross-link formation and development of parallel fiber configuration in new collagen tissue. Studies done on continuous passive motion machines have shown that movement does decrease the formation of capsular adhesions. More aggressive manipulation techniques are thought to break adhesions in the joint capsule and in the synovial folds. Manipulation also theoretically increases the length of capsular fibers. It also has been shown to break intracapsular fibrofatty adhesions. All of these responses to manipulation will have the effect of increasing the amount of arthrokinematic motion at a joint.

Inflammation produces hypertrophy of the synovial lining of the joint, due to an invasion of connective tissue fibers. This results in fibrosis of the synovial lining, which produces joint contractures. Immobilization and inflammation almost always occur concurrently. Because of this, and due to the similarity between the two responses, much of the theory behind the rationale for treating the result of immobilization with joint manipulation techniques is applicable to the treatment of joint hypomobility due to inflammation. Thus, for the joint exhibiting the sequelae of inflammation, joint manipulation lengthens thickened capsular tissue and reduces capsular adhesions.

Although theoretically the one structure being affected by joint manipulation techniques is the joint capsule, in reality it is impossible to isolate the techniques to this tissue. All periarticular tissue, including muscles, tendons, and fascia, are affected by joint manipulation techniques.

To more clearly understand the nature of soft tissue extensibility and its relation to stretching techniques, it is important to become familiar with the characteristics of the stress-strain curve (Fig 1–1). Rules of stress-strain, or load deformation, are applicable to all solid tissue. As an external tensile force is applied to a tissue (stress), the tissue goes through several transitions (strain). The first stage is the elastic phase, in which the stretched tissue returns to its original configuration once the external force is removed. The second stage is the plastic phase, where permanent elongation of the stretched tissue occurs when the external force is removed. The third stage is the failure or breaking point, in which separation of the elongated tissue occurs. Within the plastic phase, there is a point at which a decrease in load is accompanied by an increase in deformation. This is called the necking point, and is an indication that the breaking point is about to be reached. Joint manipulation techniques designed to increase extensibility of joint and periarticular tissue should be forceful enough to bring the tissue into the plastic phase but not to the breaking point. If while manipulating a joint the clinician perceives that a decrease in force is associated with a relatively large amount of deformation, this is a sign that the tissue being stretched has reached the necking point and is about to reach the breaking point. When this is felt by the clinician, the technique immediately should be terminated. The exception to this is when the goal is to break adhesions, in which case the force should be maintained until the breaking point has been reached.

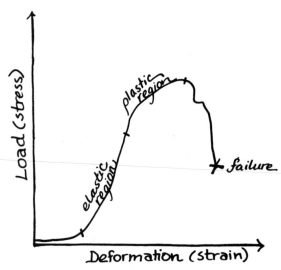

FIG 1–1.
Stress-strain curve.

There are other factors that influence the amount of joint extensibility gained through application of a manipulation technique besides the amount of force applied to a joint capsule. The speed with which the technique is administered also will determine the amount of extensibility gained; more rapidly administered techniques yield greater gains in extensibility and also are more effective in breaking adhesions. A stretch administered into the plastic phase for a long period will yield a greater amount of extensibility than a stretch administered over a short period. This accommodation to the stretched position is called "creep." The number of repetitions administered also will have an effect on the amount of extensibility gained.

As the clinician moves a joint structure through its range of accessory motion, several palpable barriers to obtaining additional motion are felt. These barriers are caused by limitations in the extensibility of joint capsular structures, as well as skin, fascia, and muscle. The first barrier corresponds to the point at which an increase in resistance is first felt and is associated with the beginning of the plastic phase of the stress-strain curve. A clinician thus can determine by palpation when articular structures are being stretched. This barrier to further motion is called the first tissue stop, end feel, or motion barrier. All joint manipulation techniques designed to increase joint extensibility must be sufficiently aggressive to take the joint through the first tissue stop. The second palpable barrier to motion corresponds to the physiologic limitation to joint play, and is called the second tissue stop (Fig 1–2). If accessory motion is restricted, joint play assessment will reveal a reduction in the amount of joint excursion before each barrier is met.

Taking a joint through its physiologic range of motion also elicits barriers. The first barrier is the end of active range of motion. The second barrier is the end of passive range of motion and corresponds to the beginning of the plastic stage. The third barrier is the physiologic limit to motion. As with joint play, if restrictions in range of motion are present, all barriers will be met sooner in the range of motion.

One of the goals of joint manipulation is to correct arthrokinematic restrictions, whereas range of motion is designed to correct osteokinematic restrictions. Often arthrokinematic limitations cause at least some of the restrictions in range of motion, and treating the arthrokinematic limitations will result in an increase in range of motion. Conversely, arthrokinematic limitations can be present in the absence of range of motion deficits. When this occurs the limitations in joint play can affect the quality of joint movement. This alteration in the quality of movement can cause joint dysfunction. For example, full shoulder elevation can occur de-

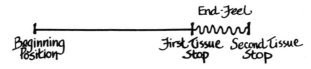

FIG 1–2.
Motion barriers with joint play.

spite inability of the humeral head to fully glide in a caudal direction in the glenoid cavity; however, this can produce impingement of suprahumeral tissue whenever the shoulder is elevated, resulting in shoulder pain.

Correcting Positional Faults

Joint surfaces can alter their position in relation to one another. If the positional abnormality is severe, it is called a subluxation; however, if minimal it is considered a positional fault. Even minimal displacement can place abnormal stress on periarticular structures and thus can be a source of pain. Manipulation of one of the joint surfaces in the direction consistent with realigning it into proper position is thought to normalize the static positioning of one joint surface in relation to the other, thus reducing pain. The technique must be aggressive enough to produce an alteration in the alignment of the two joint surfaces. For example, occasionally the lunate becomes positioned in a volar direction in relation to the radius. This often results from a fall on an outstretched arm. Treatment is directed toward manipulating the lunate in a dorsal direction in relation to the radius, resulting in restoration of normal alignment of the two articular surfaces. Positional faults are especially common in the spine.

Nutrition

Articular surfaces are avascular and receive their nutrition from synovial fluid. For diffusion of nutrients to occur, the synovial fluid must circulate within the capsule to allow nutrients to be in contact with the articular surface. Joint movement through functional activities provides a mechanism for the circulation of synovial fluid in the normal joint. Joints that are restricted often cannot obtain adequate nutrition because of insufficient range of motion to produce movement of synovial fluid within the synovial cavity. Joint manipulation techniques are thought to produce movement of fluid within the synovium. If functional mobility is also a goal of the manipulation technique being performed, the restoration of functional range of motion will aid in delivering nutrients to intracapsular tissue on a more permanent basis through active movement. Finally, movement of synovial fluid produces a decrease in the viscosity of the fluid, thus temporarily promoting greater ease in both synovial fluid movement and joint motion.

All types of manipulation techniques are capable of increasing movement of fluid within the joint.

Pain Control/Muscle Relaxation

Manipulation decreases pain in joint and periarticular structures by stimulating joint receptors. This reduces pain perception by producing blockage of pain impulses through the gate control mechanism and by producing reflexive muscle relaxation. Pain also can be decreased temporarily in certain conditions by decreasing the compressive forces on the joint. This is accomplished when techniques designed to distract the two joint surfaces are used.

Gating of pain impulses occurs when movement of periarticular tissue being manipulated stimulates fast-conducting large-diameter proprioceptive nerve fibers that block the transmission of slow-conducting small-diameter pain fibers, thus minimizing the transmission of pain impulses to the brain. Reducing pain can have a secondary effect on muscle relaxation.

Relaxation of periarticular muscles also is achieved by the stimulation of joint receptors with joint manipulation techniques. Joint receptors function to protect the joint from damage incurred by going beyond the physiologic range of motion. They also are partly responsible for determining the appropriate balance between synergistic and antagonistic muscular forces and for generating an image of body positioning and movement within the central nervous system. There are four types of joint receptors.

Type 1: Postural.
a. Stimulus
  (1) Changing mechanical stresses in the joint capsule.
  (2) May be more active with traction techniques than with oscillations.
  (3) May be activated by the presence of positional faults.
b. Characteristics
  (1) Low threshold.
  (2) Slow adapting (acts up to 1 minute following the initial stimulation).
c. Response
  (1) Gives the patient a sense of both static and dynamic position and a sense of direction amplitude and velocity of movement.
  (2) Produces increased tone in the muscle being stretched and relaxation in the muscle antagonistic to that being stretched.
d. Location
  (1) Located in the superficial capsule.
  (2) Located primarily in the neck, hip, and shoulder.

Type 2: Dynamic.
a. Stimulus.
  (1) Sudden changes in joint motion.
  (2) May be more active with oscillation techniques than with traction.
b. Characteristics.
  (1) Low threshold.
  (2) Rapid adapting (acts for ½ second following each motion).
c. Response.
  (1) Gives the patient a sense of joint acceleration and deceleration.
  (2) Produces increased tone in the muscle being stretched and relaxation in the muscle antagonistic to the one being stretched when the joint is at the end of range.
d. Location.
  (1) Located in the deep layers of ligaments and capsule.
  (2) Located primarily in the lumbar spine, hand, foot, jaw.

Type 3: Inhibitive.
a. Stimulus.
  (1) Stretch at end of range.
b. Characteristics.
  (1) High threshold.
  (2) Very slow adapting (acts for several minutes following the initial stimulation).
  (3) More active with fast manipulation techniques.
c. Response.
  (1) Gives the patient a sense of dynamic movement and direction of movement.
  (2) Inhibits muscle tone.
d. Location.
  (1) Located primarily in joint ligaments.

Type 4. Nociceptive.
a. Stimulus.
  (1) Marked mechanical deformation or tension.
  (2) Direct mechanical or chemical irritation.
b. Characteristics.
  (1) High threshold.
  (2) Nonadapting.
c. Response.
  (1) Produces tonic muscle contraction.
d. Location.
  (1) Located in most tissues.

When treating a patient for the purpose of relaxing the musculature surrounding the joint, the direction of the technique should be such that the capsular structures opposite the musculature to be relaxed are stretched. This will result in contraction of the musculature adjacent to the stretched capsular tissue and relaxation of antagonist muscles. If oscillations, or treatments directed parallel to the joint surface, are being used, the direction of the oscillation should be opposite that which would increase joint play in the capsule adjacent to the muscle being relaxed. If the goal also is to increase extensibility of periarticular structures, the manipulation should be directed opposite that which would decrease the restriction, to relax the musculature limiting motion, and then in the direction that will treat the restriction in order to increase extensibility. Treating with oscillations may be more effective in producing relaxation in the lumbar spine, hand, foot, and jaw.

If traction, or treatments directed perpendicular to the joint surface, are being used for relaxation purposes, the joint should be positioned so that the capsular stretch occurs in the part of the capsule opposite the muscle being relaxed. The restricted range therefore should be avoided. If the neck, hip, or shoulder are being treated for relaxation, traction may be more effective than oscillations.

Joint manipulation can be used to relax joints exhibiting excessive movement if the techniques are limited to those that do not bring the joint through the first tissue stop. Techniques that bring the joint through the first tissue stop are appropriate only if indicated for other reasons. If so, thrust manipulations are especially effective in promoting relaxation, because they stimulate the type 3 receptors.

Meniscoid Impingement

An intracapsular meniscoid structure has been shown to exist within the facet joints of the spine. This structure can become caught between the two facet joint surfaces, causing locking of the two joint surfaces accompanied by pain. Joint manipulation techniques, particularly procedures involving gapping of the two joint surfaces, are believed to release the meniscoid tissue and to restore normal motion to the vertebrae affected.

Reduction of Disc Herniation

Some clinicians believe that spinal disc herniations can be treated by spinal manipulation, especially thrust manipulation techniques. It has been hypothesized that during spinal manipulation sufficient negative pressure is created in the space between the vertebral bodies to draw the disc material back into the intervertebral space. To date this concept has not been substantiated. Thrust manipulations generally are chosen to accomplish this goal.

Psychologic Benefits

One must not discount the psychologic benefit to a patient of a treatment composed of techniques requiring touch. This is especially true in a medical system in which few practitioners remain who heal by the laying on of hands.

PRECAUTIONS

Joint manipulation should not be performed in the presence of the following conditions.

1. Any undiagnosed lesion
2. Joint ankylosis
3. Joint hypermobility, if techniques that take the joint through the first tissue stop are being considered, unless a positional fault is being treated.

In the Spine:

1. Any indication of vertebrobasilar insufficiency in the upper cervical spine if the cervical spine is being treated, because joint manipulation has been known to produce cerebral vascular accidents
2. Rheumatoid arthritis in the cervical spine if the cervical spine is being treated, because joint manipulation may produce dislocation of upper cervical joints
3. Traumatized upper cervical ligaments if the cervical spine is being treated, because joint manipulation may result in dislocation of the upper cervical joints
4. Cauda equina syndrome if the lumbar spine is being treated, because manipulation may exacerbate the condition.

In any of the following conditions, the clinician should carefully consider whether the benefits outweigh the risks of performing joint manipulation techniques. This is especially true with the more aggressive techniques.

1. An infection in the area being treated
2. Malignancy in the area being treated
3. An unhealed fracture in the area being treated
4. Inflammatory arthritis in the area being treated, especially if in a state of exacerbation
5. Metabolic bone diseases, such as osteoporosis, Paget disease, and tuberculosis
6. Any debilitating disease that compromises the integrity of periarticular tissue, such as advanced diabetes
7. Considerable joint effusion in the area being treated, since it is difficult to obtain an accurate assessment of joint extensibility because swelling already has taken up much of the slack in the joint capsule
8. Considerable joint irritability or pain in the area being treated
9. Protective muscle spasm to the extent that the clinician is unable to assess mobility in the area being treated
10. Pain in adjacent segments that is aggravated by the placement of the clinician's hands when attempting to perform manipulation techniques

In the Spine:

1. Spinal cord involvement in the area being treated
2. Spondylolisthesis in the area being treated
3. Severe scoliosis in the area being treated
4. Suspected spinal aneurysm in the area being treated
5. Pregnancy, if the lumbar spine or pelvis is being treated, because it may induce labor
6. Positive neurologic signs if the spine or pelvis is being treated with thrust techniques
7. Genetic disorders affecting the spine, such as Down syndrome when cervical spine treatments are being considered

ASSESSMENT

All patients should undergo a full evaluation before any treatment is performed, including treatment with joint manipulation. An evaluation should comprise a complete history and a physical examination including inspection, palpation, range of motion assessment, joint play assessment, neurologic assessment, strength assessment, and any appropriate special tests. Radiographs should be examined when available. Signs and symptoms should be consistent with the diagnosis, and a complete plan of care should be generated, taking into consideration the diagnosis, the factors contributing to the physical dysfunction, the patient's goals, the extent of the injury, and any medical concerns.

Assessment of joint play is critical to the performance of any joint manipulation technique. Joint play assessment is initiated by placing the patient in the resting, or loose-packed, position. This is the joint position in which the ligaments are most lax and there is the most distance between the two articular surfaces. In all joints, both these conditions occur simultaneously in one position. The resting position also is usually the position adopted by a joint in dysfunction as the position of most comfort. Joints are tested in the resting position because this is the position with the greatest amount of joint play. If limitations in range of motion or pain prevent the clinician from placing the joint in the resting position, then the position most closely approximating the resting position should be used. This is called the actual resting position. The resting position for all of the joints are listed in the introductory section of the chapter for each joint.

Joint play is assessed by moving one of the articular surfaces of the joint in a direction that is either parallel or perpendicular to the joint. These directions are determined by first identifying the concave joint surface and visualizing the plane of that joint surface as if the joint surface were flattened out. This plane is called the treatment plane. Since the treatment plane is identified in reference to the concave joint surface, it moves if the concave joint surface is part of the moving bone, and stays stationary if the convex joint surface moves. Passively moving either bone in a direction perpendicular to the treatment plane constitutes a traction or distraction joint play assessment, and moving either bone in a direction parallel to the treatment plane constitutes an oscillation or a gliding joint play assessment (Fig 1–3). It is important to recognize that because of this relationship, traction manipulations administered to a long bone are not always performed along the long axis of that bone. For example, because of the ventral angulation of the forearm in relation to the treatment plane of the ulna, humeroulnar traction manipulations are performed in a direction of 45 degrees less flexion than the angle of the forearm (Fig 1–4,A and B), because this is the direction perpendicular to the treatment plane. Traction manipulations directed along the axis of the long bone are called long axis distractions, to distinguish them from tractions administered perpendicular to the

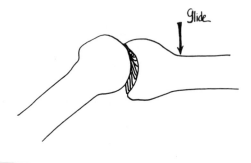

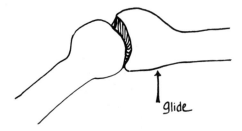

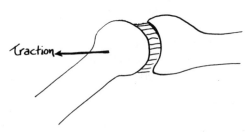

FIG 1–3.
Glides and traction.

treatment plane. In general, correctly identifying the orientation of the concave joint surface is necessary for the accurate execution of the evaluation or treatment manipulation.

Joint play assessment entails evaluation of the amount of excursion present in a particular joint when moved in a particular direction, evaluation of the presence of pain, and determination of the type of resistance felt at the end of the range for joint play. Excursion is determined by comparing the joint with the same joint on the opposite side, assuming this joint is not in dysfunction. If no "normal" joint exists, then joint excursion must be determined by comparison with the clinician's experience with evaluating the same joint on oneself or in other patients. Joint excursion is evaluated by performing either a glide or a traction manipulation and by moving the bone up to the end of the available range. Thus an assessment glide is a movement of one bone parallel to the treatment plane with enough excursion to go up to and slightly through the first tissue stop. This corresponds to a grade 3 treatment glide (see Treatment). An assessment traction is a distraction perpendicular to the treatment plane with enough excursion to go up to and slightly through the first tissue stop. This corresponds to a grade 2 to grade 3 treatment traction (also described under Treatment). The first tissue stop is felt by the clinician as an increase in the resistance as one bone is moved on the other bone. It

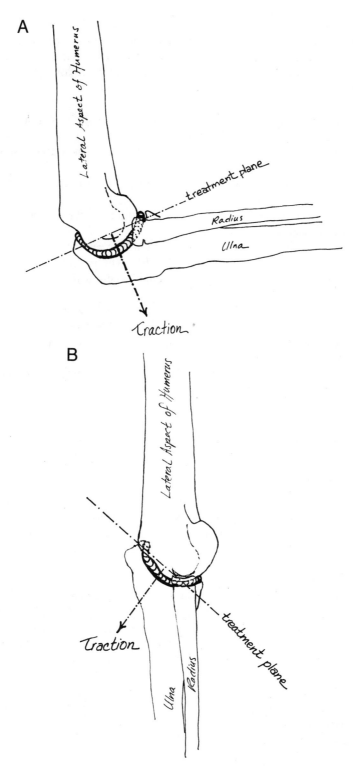

FIG 1–4.
Treatment planes. **A,** humeroulnar traction at 90 degrees of flexion. **B,** humeroulnar traction at 0 degrees.

also corresponds with the end of the elastic phase and the beginning of the plastic phase on the stress-strain curve. The amount of motion from the resting position of the two joint surfaces to the first tissue stop is graded according to the amount of excursion the bone undergoes before reaching the first tissue stop. This can be graded according to the following scale, and has the following treatment implications.

Grade 0: There is no motion between the two articulating surfaces. Manipulation is not indicated, and surgery should be considered.

Grade 1: There is considerable limitation between the two joint surfaces. Manipulation is indicated.

Grade 2: There is a slight limitation between the two joint surfaces. Manipulation is indicated.

Grade 3: The amount of movement between the two joint surfaces is normal. Manipulation is not indicated to increase joint extensibility.

Grade 4: There is a slight increase in the excursion between the two joint surfaces. Manipulation is not indicated to increase joint extensibility. The patient should be treated with stabilization through exercise and/or taping, and should be educated regarding correct posture and positions to avoid.

Grade 5: There is a considerable increase in the excursion between the two joint surfaces. Manipulation is not indicated to increase joint extensibility. The patient should be treated with stabilization through exercise and bracing, and should be educated regarding correct posture and positions to avoid.

Grade 6: The joint is unstable. Manipulation is not indicated to increase joint extensibility. Surgery should be considered.

An alternative grading scale consists of three categories. In this system, grades 0, 1, and 2 are grouped together and labeled "hypomobile"; grade 3 is considered "normal"; and grades 4, 5, and 6 are labeled "hypermobile." This scale has the advantage of being more reliable because there are fewer categories.

It also is important to assess whether pain is present when evaluating joint play with oscillation and traction techniques. Pain in conjunction with hypomobility indicates an acute sprain with guarding or an inflamed joint. In these circumstances, it is important to consider whether what appears to be hypomobility is in fact muscle guarding and if the muscle guarding is masking a hypermobile condition. If so, joint manipulation may be detrimental. Hypomobility without pain indicates a chronic adhesion or contracture. Manipulation techniques that bring the joint through the first tissue stop are indicated in this situation. Normal mobility with pain indicates a mild sprain without disruption of capsular fibers. Joint manipulation for stretching of periarticular structures is not indicated in the presence of normal mobility, but the patient may benefit from gentle techniques to provide nutrition to intra-articular structures, decrease pain, promote normal alignment of collagen fibers, and prevent restrictions in joint play. Normal mobility without pain indicates an absence of joint dysfunction. Excessive mobility with pain indicates a partial sprain of capsular tissues; excessive mobility without pain indicates a complete sprain of capsular tissues. In both instances stabilization techniques are indicated. When pain accompanies hypermobility, gentle manipulations can be used to decrease pain and promote joint nutrition.

End feels also are assessed during the evaluation of joint play. Joint play end feels are either bony or firm. A bony end feel indicates that either there is bony hypertrophy in the joint blocking additional motion or that the restrictions in the joint capsule are causing the two articulating surfaces to jam together. A firm end feel indicates that soft tissue is limiting further motion. Some clinicians can delineate between joint and muscular soft tissue restrictions by assessing the type of firm end feel.

Identifying positional faults also is an integral component of the assessment. The clinician must determine during the palpation component of the evaluation process whether the joint surfaces are aligned appropriately to one another. Once an alteration in alignment is suspected, the clinician then must assess whether the perceived malalignment is a positional fault or a bony abnormality. Positional faults are confirmed by determining that joint play movement in the direction of the positional fault is less than movement opposite the direction of the positional fault, and that either movement into the positional fault, movement to correct the positional fault, or both are associated with a reproduction of the patient's symptoms. Thus evaluation of a volar positional fault of the lunate on the radius would result in a decrease of further volar gliding of the lunate on the radius, and either volar or dorsal gliding would reproduce the patient's symptoms.

Compression and distraction of the two articular surfaces of a joint also are assessed for response to pain. If pain increases with compression and is relieved with distraction, this indicates possible involvement of the articular surface. On the other hand, if pain is relieved with compression and increased with traction, the pain may be capsular or ligamentous.

When performing an assessment manipulation, the clinician should keep the following principles in mind:

1. The patient should exhibit no muscle guarding and should be as relaxed as possible.

2. The clinician should be efficient with body mechanics, and should stand with a wide base of support. The manipulating force should be as close to the clinician's center of gravity as possible. The force ideally should be directed downward. If a downward force is not feasible, a horizontally directed force should be attempted. This is especially true when treating larger joints, but is less important when evaluating the smaller joints of the hand and the foot. The clinician should use his or her weight to assist with the force of manipulation whenever possible.

3. The joint should be tested in the resting position if the patient is capable of attaining that position. If not, the joint should be tested in the actual resting position.

4. The clinician's grasp should be firm yet painless.

5. One bone should be stabilized with the clinician's hand or other body part, a belt, a wedge, or the treatment table.

6. The other bone is manipulated with the clinician's hand.

7. Both the stabilizing force and the manipulating force should be as close to the joint surface as possible, to control the motion as closely as possible.

8. The patient's pain should be monitored during the assessment, and appropriate modifications should be made based on the pain response.

9. Accessory motion should be assessed by comparison with the corresponding joint on the other side of the body, whenever possible.

10. Only one movement should be performed at a time. For example, the clinician should not manipulate a bone into dorsal glide from a ventrally glided position, because it is more difficult to assess movement in this manner.

11. Only one joint should be manipulated at a time.

12. Each technique is both an evaluative technique and a treatment technique; therefore the clinician continually evaluates during treatment. Formal assessments also should be made before and after treatment.

Joints are capable of several types of joint motion. Spinning is one type of joint motion (Fig 1–5). Spinning is a movement of one bone on the other such that one point on both bones remains in contact with the other, and the rest of the articular surface of one bone rotates in relation to the other. Rolling is another type of motion (Fig 1–6), which occurs when one point on one bone comes into contact with a point on the other bone that is equidistant

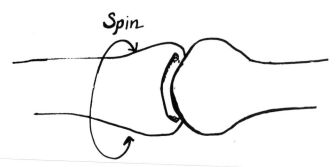

FIG 1–5.
Spin.

from the original contact point. Sliding is the third type of motion (Fig 1–7), and occurs when one point on one bone stays in contact with the articulating surface of the other bone but at a new point. Rolling and spinning are restored primarily with passive range of motion, although restoring the arthrokinematic motion in all directions will be of some assistance in restoring rolling and spinning motion. Sliding is the predominant motion to be restored by joint manipulation techniques.

The direction of the slide should correspond with a specific physiologic movement and depends on the shape of the articular surface. Most joints are composed of a convex surface articulating with a reciprocally shaped concave surface. If the concave surface is the moving surface, the direction of the slide is the same as the physiologic movement. If the convex surface is the moving surface the direction of the slide is opposite that of the physiologic movement (Fig 1–8). The direction of force imparted with the evaluation oscillation therefore corresponds to a specific physiologic movement based on the concave-convex relationship of the joint surfaces. For example, if a concave tibia moves on a convex femur, as in open kinematic chain activities, the tibia glides in the same direction as the physiologic motion. If a convex femur moves on a concave tibia, as in closed kinematic chain activities, the femur glides in a direction opposite that of the physiologic motion. Range of motion limitations should correspond to the limitation in joint play based on concave-convex rules. Thus limitations in knee flexion should correspond to a decrease in joint play of the tibia gliding dorsally on the femur or of the femur gliding ventrally on the tibia. Concave-convex rules are difficult to apply to joints in which the articulation is not at the end of the bone, such as the radioulnar joint, because the motion to be analyzed is the motion of the bony surface opposite the joint surface, and this movement is often difficult to follow. In addition, bones that move primarily by sliding and that have relatively flat articular surfaces, such as the facet joints of the spine, tend to slide in the direction of the physiologic motion regardless of the concave-convex joint surface relationship.

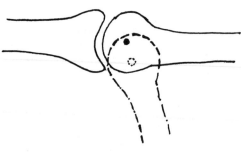

FIG 1–6.
Roll.

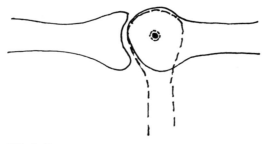

FIG 1–7.
Slide.

Ovoid joints are shaped such that one joint surface is concave in its entirety. This joint surface articulates with a joint surface that is convex in its entirety (Fig 1–9). Sellar joints are shaped such that one joint surface is concave in one direction and convex in the direction perpendicular to the concave surface. The articulating joint surface is reciprocally convex to match the concave surface of its adjoining articulation, and concave in the direction perpendicular to the convex surface (Fig 1–10). The two articulating surfaces therefore are congruent. The moving bone slides in the same direction as the physiologic movement in one plane

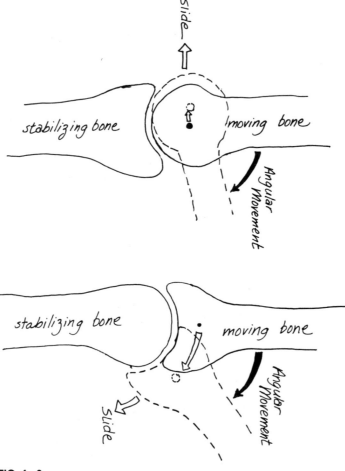

FIG 1–8.
Concave-convex rules.

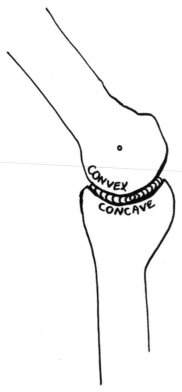

FIG 1–9.
Ovoid joint.

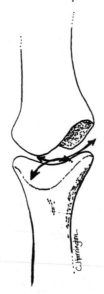

FIG 1–10.
Sellar joint.

of motion and opposite the direction of the physiologic movement in the perpendicular plane.

Articular surfaces are not entirely congruent with one another. Motion therefore is never pure, and motion in one plane often is associated with a specific pattern of motion in at least one other plane. This phenomenon is called conjugate motion or coupled motion. Limitations in one movement often occur in conjunction with limitations in the motion to which that movement is coupled. Other factors that may contribute to the presence of coupled motion include muscular and ligamentous control of motion.

When the entire joint is traumatized, the capsule of each joint undergoes a characteristic pattern of restriction, which is specific for each joint and which can be detected when evaluating passive range of motion. This pattern of restriction is called the capsular pattern. If passive range of motion of a joint is limited in this characteristic pattern of restriction, this indicates that the dysfunction involves the entire joint capsule. Examples of dysfunctions involving the entire joint capsule include osteoarthritic and traumatic arthritic conditions. Joint conditions that do not necessarily cause a capsular pattern of restrictions include such diagnoses as meniscal problems and ligamentous sprains. Capsular patterns are important when diagnosing, because the presence of a capsular pattern would indicate that the diagnosis must be one in which the entire joint capsule is involved. Capsular patterns of restriction for all of the joints are listed in the introduction section of the chapter for each joint, in order of restriction from greatest to least. Movements not listed are irrelevant to the identification of the capsular pattern.

TREATMENT

Treatment manipulations are graded according to the amount of excursion imparted to the joint. Traction treatment manipulations are graded as follows (Fig 1–11).

Grade 1: Slow, small amplitude movement perpendicular to the concave joint surface that does not take the joint up to the first tissue stop.
Grade 2: Slow, larger amplitude movement perpendicular to the concave joint surface that takes the joint up to the first tissue stop.
Grade 3: Slow, even larger amplitude movement perpendicular to the concave joint surface that takes the joint up to and slightly through the first tissue stop.

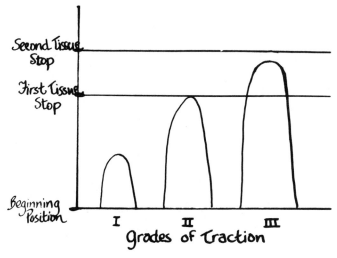

FIG 1–11.
Grades of traction.

Grades 1 and 2 are used for pain reduction, while grade 3 is used to reduce pain, increase periarticular extensibility, correct positional faults, and reduce spinal disc herniations. All grades of traction increase nutrition to articular structures.

Treatment oscillation manipulations also are graded (Fig 1–12). Glides are graded along a scale of 1 to 5 as follows:

Grade 1: Slow, small-amplitude oscillatory movement parallel to the concave joint surface that does not take the joint up to the first tissue stop.

Grade 2: Slow, larger-amplitude oscillatory movement parallel to the concave joint surface that does not take the joint up to the first tissue stop.

Grade 3: Slow, large-amplitude oscillatory movement parallel to the concave joint surface that takes the joint up to and slightly through the first tissue stop.

Grade 4: Slow, small-amplitude oscillatory movement parallel to the concave joint surface that takes the joint up to and slightly through the first tissue stop.

Grade 5: Fast, small-amplitude, high-velocity nonoscillatory movement parallel to the concave joint surface that begins at the first tissue stop and then takes the joint through the first tissue stop, also called a thrust manipulation.

All treatment oscillations are performed with at least grade 1 traction when feasible to decrease compression of joint surfaces. Grades 1 and 2 oscillations are used for pain reduction. Grades 3 and 4 are used to reduce pain, increase periarticular extensibility, correct positional faults, and release impinged meniscoid tissue in the spine. All grades of oscillation increase nutrition to articular structures. Grade 5 oscillations are used to reduce spinal disc herniations, and also are appropriate when grades 3 and 4 have failed to accomplish the goal of treatment. Since joint manipulation techniques can traumatize joints, the risk always exists that a particular technique can result in an increase rather than a decrease in joint restrictions. The clinician therefore always should use the least aggressive technique required to accomplish the goal of treatment.

One method of determining how aggressively a patient can be treated is by examining the pattern of pain to resistance with the passive range of motion corresponding to the particular manipulation technique being considered. If pain occurs before resistance is met with passive range of motion, then grades 1 and 2 oscillation techniques and grades 1 and 2 traction techniques are indicated to treat pain so that the patient will be able to tolerate a more complete

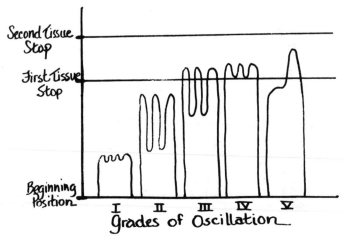

FIG 1–12.
Grades of oscillation.

evaluation. If pain occurs at the same point in the range of motion as the first barrier to motion, then the patient should be able to tolerate up to grade 3 oscillations and tractions. If pain occurs after the first barrier to motion is met or if no pain occurs with overpressure beyond the first motion barrier, the patient should be able to tolerate up to grade 3 tractions and grades 4 and 5 oscillations.

Much debate exists as to whether to treat with techniques designed to increase joint mobility in the presence of any pain that occurs with joint play testing. In this book, the approach is taken that if the joint is restricted, and if that restriction is considered to be a component of the dysfunction, then the restriction should be treated. If a positional fault is present and is considered to be a component of the dysfunction, then the positional fault should be corrected. The same is true for meniscoid impingements. This holds true regardless of the pattern of pain presented with joint play testing. A thorough examination and diagnosis of the dysfunction are therefore crucial in determining an appropriate treatment regimen that includes joint manipulation techniques. It often is helpful to use techniques designed to treat the pain and irritation before and after performing the technique required to resolve the dysfunction. On occasion, treatment of pain may take several treatment sessions before the patient can tolerate the technique designed to treat the dysfunction.

This philosophy contradicts that of Maitland, who advocates manipulating in the direction of reproducible symptoms, and Maigne who advocates always moving the joint in a pain-free direction.

There are several methods of treating joint dysfunction caused by restrictions or positional faults with manipulation. The direct technique is the most common form of joint manipulation. In the direct technique, the joint is moved passively using oscillation or traction techniques. The techniques used to treat a joint in dysfunction are the same techniques as those used to assess joint play. Restrictions are treated with the same assessment manipulation that identified the restriction. The restriction should be consistent with the corresponding loss of physiologic motion, based on the concave-convex rules. Positional faults are treated with techniques that manipulate the bone into its normal alignment.

The direct technique should be initiated with the joint in the resting position. This is the safest position in which to treat, because compressive forces are minimal, and the patient's response can be observed before proceeding to more aggressive positions. Most of the techniques discussed in this book are described in the resting position, because this is the safest position and because it allows for the greatest amount of joint excursion. It is important to realize, however, that although this position is the safest, it usually is not the most effective position in which to treat, if the goal is to increase joint extensibility. The periarticular tissue that is limiting normal joint motion is most stretched when the joint is positioned as close to the restricted range as pain will allow.

Manipulations never should be performed in the close-packed position. This is the position of maximal congruency of articular surfaces and the position in which the ligaments are on maximal stretch. Close-packed positioning produces too much compressive force on the articulating surfaces. If the close-packed position can be achieved, there is minimal, if any, restriction in the joint capsule to be restored. Close-packed positions for all of the joints are listed in the introductory section for each joint.

Close-packed positioning occasionally is used to minimize unwanted motion at an adjacent joint. For example, it might be advantageous to place the elbow in the close-packed position for the humeroulnar joint when manipulating the humeroradial joint, to minimize unwanted humeroulnar motion. In the spine, motion at adjacent joints often is minimized by positioning the spine so that the adjacent joints are at the end of their available range. The close-packed position seldom is used in the spine, because this position is end-range backward bending and is not comfortable for most patients. However, the principle is similar to that of close packing in that both techniques prevent motion at adjacent joints.

Muscle energy is a specific type of direct technique using voluntary contraction of the patient's muscles. The joint is placed in a specific position to facilitate optimal contraction of a particular muscle or muscle group. The patient then is asked to contract that muscle or muscle group against counterpressure, causing the muscle to contract isometrically. This causes the muscle to pull on the bony attachment that is not being stabilized by the clinician, thus moving one bone in relation to its articulating counterpart. The articulating counterpart must be stabilized for this to occur. The muscle contraction should be isometric, with the intensity of the contraction controlled by the clinician. The contraction therefore occurs in a precisely controlled direction with a precisely controlled joint position in all three planes, and requires a distinctly executed counterforce. All of these conditions are the responsibility of the clinician, rendering most muscle energy techniques difficult for a beginner to execute. Most isometric contractions are held for 3 to 7 seconds, and techniques are repeated approximately three times before reassessment.

Muscle energy techniques have the advantage of allowing the patient to control the manipulation; thus if too much pain is reproduced during the maneuver the patient can terminate the procedure. Muscle energy also can be used to strengthen muscle and to lengthen contractile tissue. The technique for this rationale is called "hold relax" by Knott and Voss.[3] The technique is thought to work by resetting the gain in the muscle spindles. It has been hypothesized that muscles surrounding a positional fault or a joint that is restricted have undergone length-tension changes consistent with the altered positioning of the articular surfaces or the restrictions in range of motion. Muscle energy therefore is an extremely valuable technique for correcting positional faults or joint hypomobility because the technique combines methods to increase extensibility of periarticular tissue with methods to restore a length-tension relationship to muscles controlling joint motion and position consistent with maintaining that joint in a normally functioning state.

Another approach to treatment is the indirect technique. In this approach the joint is treated in the direction opposite the direction of the restriction. It is believed that joint restrictions can be caused by jamming of the two articular surfaces. To release the jammed surfaces the manipulation should occur in the direction opposite the restriction, in much the same way that someone would first close a door that is stuck in order to open it. It is advisable to try this technique in situations in which direct techniques have been shown to be ineffective.

Oscillations generally are performed at a rate of about two to three per second for about 1 minute, followed by a rest period of several seconds. Traction techniques are held for about 10 seconds, followed by a rest period of several seconds. Both are performed for up to several minutes before reassessing for appropriateness of continuing the treatment. Typically, several manipulation techniques are performed per treatment session, and treatment sessions can take 5 to 45 minutes. Manipulations always are performed in conjunction with other treatment techniques. If pain is a component of the patient's problem other techniques may include modalities, such as heat, ice, and/or electrical stimulation, rest, bracing, and patient education. If reduction of joint restrictions is the primary goal of treatment, adjunct techniques may include range of motion and strengthening exercises, proprioceptive neuromuscular facilitation (PNF) hold relax and contract relax techniques, soft tissue mobilization, and patient education.

Treatment directed at increasing joint extensibility, correcting positional faults, and releasing impinged meniscoid tissue often involve trauma to periarticular structures. The patient therefore can expect to experience soreness after treatment. If the patient does not have soreness after treatment, then more aggressive techniques can be initiated if indicated. If the patient has soreness for between 4 and 12 hours after treatment, then the clinician should continue to treat using techniques that are as aggressive as those previously used, because this is an appropriate response to manipulation treatments. If the patient experiences an increase in symptoms for more than 12 hours after treatment or experiences swelling or muscle guarding in the area of the joint being treated, then either the wrong technique was performed or the treatment was too aggressive. In such instances reevaluation is indicated. In general, the patient should be reevaluated often to ascertain that the nature of the problem has not changed and goals are being reached.

Treatment sessions should be at least 48 hours apart to allow the patient to recover from any ill effects of the previous treatment. Treatment should be terminated once all goals have been reached or if gains in function have reached a plateau.

Little research has been done on the efficacy of joint manipulation techniques. Much of the research that has been performed has been on spinal manipulation. In general, the studies have concluded that spinal manipulation improves outcome in the short term but has no significant long-term value. Most of the studies that have been performed on extremity joints have centered around the efficacy of manipulation under anesthesia, and response to treatment with manipulation was compared with the patient's status before manipulation. In these studies, outcome generally was positive. One study that analyzed the effect of joint manipulation on range of motion of the metacarpophalangeal joint was performed in nonanesthetized patients following immobilization for a fracture. Results suggest that joint manipulation does increase range of motion.[4] Clearly, additional research is needed to more clearly delineate the rationale behind the use of manipulation as a treatment technique and the efficacy of treatment with manipulation in different patient populations.

REFERENCES

1. Funk IK: *New Standard Dictionary of the English Language.* New York, Funk & Wagnalls, 1963.
2. Greenman PE: *Principles of Manual Medicine,* Baltimore, Williams & Wilkins, 1989.
3. Knott M, Voss DE: Proprioceptive neuromuscular facilitation, ed 2, New York, Harper & Row, 1968.
4. Randall T, Partner L, Haus BA: Effects of joint mobilization on joint stiffness and acute motion of the metacarpophalangeal joint. *J Orthop Sports Phys Ther,* 16(1):30, 1992.

Figure 2 − 1_____

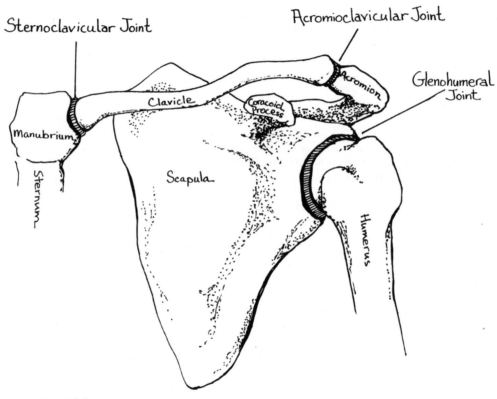

Shoulder Joints

Chapter 2

Shoulder

The primary purpose of the shoulder complex is to allow for positioning of the hand for functional activities. The shoulder complex is made up of four joints, all of which contribute to attaining full range of motion at the shoulder: the glenohumeral joint, the sternoclavicular joint, the acromioclavicular joint, and the scapulothoracic joint. Approximately 120 degrees of motion into flexion and abduction must take place at these joints for most functional activities to occur.

The glenohumeral articulation is the most mobile joint in the human body. This is achieved in part because the humeral head is much larger than its articulating counterpart, the glenoid cavity. The sole attachment of the shoulder complex to the axial skeletal system at the sternoclavicular joint also contributes to its mobility. Internal forces acting to stabilize the shoulder often are inadequate. Many disorders of the shoulder therefore can be attributable to its large arc of motion.

SCAPULAR ELEVATION

Scapulothoracic joint elevation and protraction accompany scapular elevation. Mobility at this articulation characteristically is hypermobile in patients with chronic or severe glenohumeral restrictions, resulting in alteration of the normal scapulohumeral rhythm. Scapular elevation is accompanied by a caudal glide of the clavicle on the sternum and lateral rotation of the scapula. The latter is restored with scapular cranial and lateral glides. Conversely, scapular depression is accompanied by cranial glide of the clavicle on the sternum and medial rotation of the scapula, which is restored with scapular caudal and medial glides. The clavicle glides in the frontal plane on the acromion as it elevates. There is no specific manipulation for restoring elevation and depression at the acromioclavicular joint, since only ventral and dorsal glides are feasible. In such a situation, it is appropriate to ensure that both these glides are restored, in which case arthrokinematic motion should proceed normally.

PROTRACTION AND RETRACTION

Protraction and retraction occur at the sternoclavicular, acromioclavicular, and scapulothoracic joints. Protraction is accompanied by a ventral glide of the clavicle on the sternum and a lateral glide of the scapula on the thorax; the opposite occurs with retraction.

ABDUCTION AND ADDUCTION

The glenoid is a pear-shaped biconcave joint. With abduction, the humeral head glides caudally into the lower concavity of the glenoid. The inferior folds of the joint capsule, present when the shoulder is in the anatomic position, unfold as abduction occurs. During immobilization in adduction these folds often adhere to one another. Restoring and maintaining the normal joint accessory motion of caudal gliding of the humerus on the glenoid is thought to reduce these adhesions, allowing the humeral head to glide into the inferior cavity of the glenoid with shoulder abduction.

With activities involving shoulder abduction there is some variation among individuals as to the relative amount of glenohumeral vs. scapulothoracic motion. During the first 30 degrees of motion the scapula attempts to stabilize itself against the thorax.[4, 5, 10] Although the degree of scapular motion during this "setting" phase is variable, the greater proportion of the motion occurs at the glenohumeral joint. After this phase, it generally is accepted that the glenohumeral joint moves 2 degrees for every 1 degree at the scapulothoracic joint,[4, 5, 8] although reported ratios vary from 1.25:1 to 3:1.[1] This ratio of glenohumeral to scapulothoracic motion also varies depending on whether motion was measured in the coronal plane or in the plane of the scapula, which is angulated 30 degrees ventral to the coronal plane. The scapular plane is regarded more commonly as the appropriate plane in which to measure abduction, because it more closely resembles functional movement, although goniometric measurements traditionally are performed in the coronal plane. Measurements in the scapular plane correspond to the 2:1 ratio,[9] whereas coronal plane motion tends to result in relatively less participation from the glenohumeral joint.[3] The relationship between the scapula and humerus is not linear throughout abduction beyond 30 degrees. Several patterns of scapulohumeral rhythm have been reported; however, in a majority of individuals scapular motion predominates in the middle ranges of elevation,[1, 8] and glenohumeral motion predominates at the end ranges.[3]

With shoulder abduction to 90 degrees the clavicle elevates and protracts as the the scapula elevates, protracts, and rotates laterally.[5] The clavicle elevates 4 degrees for every 10 degrees of humeral elevation.[4, 8] Most of this motion takes place at the sternoclavicular joint. After reaching 90 degrees the acromioclavicular joint becomes close packed and does not contribute to additional shoulder abduction. Additional motion into abduction occurs as the clavicle rotates dorsally on its longitudinal axis.[5] The coracoclavicular ligament is responsible for this motion in that it pulls the clavicle into rotation as the clavicle moves away from the coracoid process during elevation.[8] Because the shape of the clavicle is similar to that of a crank, clavicular rotation is accompanied by elevation of the acromion.

All of these considerations are important in determining the amount of motion to restore at each of the four joints when treating hypomobility into shoulder abduction. Caution should be used whenever manipulating the sternoclavicular, acromioclavicular, and scapulothoracic joints, because these joints also frequently are hypermobile. If they are hypermobile, to treat them inadvertently with techniques sufficiently aggressive to stretch articular structures would be detrimental.

External rotation occurs in conjunction with abduction in the coronal plane. Abduction produces twisting of the glenohumeral ligaments, which creates a tendency to external rotation at the shoulder.[5, 7] Abduction in the scapular plane does not place sufficient tension on the glenohumeral ligaments to cause external rotation, and therefore external rotation is not a component of this movement.[3, 7] In both planes of motion, combining external rotation with abduction aids elevation by bringing the greater tuberosity behind the acromial shelf, thus avoiding impingement of the two structures in the suprahumeral space.[8] It therefore is crucial to ensure that adequate external rotation is present before aggressively treating abduction restrictions. Abduction is restored by gliding the humerus caudally, and external rotation is restored by gliding it ventrally.

Ligamentous structures are primarily responsible for stabilizing the glenohumeral joint during abduction and external rotation. At rest, dislocation is prevented by the superior capsule, the coracohumeral ligament, and the supraspinatus muscle.[11] External rotation at 0 degrees of abduction is limited by the inferior glenohumeral ligament and the subscapularis.[11] The middle and inferior glenohumeral ligaments and the subscapularis limit motion in the middle ranges of abduction combined with external rotation, whereas at the extremes of abduction with external rotation, motion is limited by the inferior glenohumeral ligament.[11] These structures are also the most likely structures stretched with joint manipulation techniques to increase abduction with lateral rotation.

Adduction to neutral occurs in conjunction with humeral cranial gliding and rarely is limited. Horizontal adduction occurs in conjunction with humeral dorsal gliding, and horizontal abduction with ventral gliding. Limitations in both these directions often occur in conjunction with other limitations.

FLEXION AND EXTENSION

Flexion occurs in conjunction with internal rotation of the humerus.[2, 4, 6] This is facilitated in part by the shape of the ligamentous structures[6] and in part because musculature responsible for shoulder flexion also internally rotates the shoulder.[2] It therefore is necessary to ensure that adequate internal rotation is present before aggressively treating flexion restrictions. Flexion and internal rotation are restored by gliding the humerus dorsally. Extension to neutral rarely is limited. Hyperextension is accompanied by a ventral glide of the humerus.

Scapular and clavicular motion during flexion is similar to motion during abduction, with several exceptions. Flexion is accompanied by more scapular protraction than with abduction.[8] Scapular setting takes place during the first 60 degrees of flexion,[4, 8] after which the glenohumeral to scapulothoracic motion ratio of 2:1 ensues.[4, 8] The greater tuberosity does not obstruct the suprahumeral space with flexion, as it does with abduction.[8]

ROTATION

External rotation occurs primarily at the glenohumeral joint,[8] whereas internal rotation is accompanied by scapular retraction and associated clavicular movements. Normal internal rotation at the glenohumeral joint therefore is not possible without adequate scapular mobility.

Glenohumeral Joint

Osteokinematic degrees of freedom:	3 motions:
	Flexion/extension
	Abduction/adduction
	Internal/external rotation
Ligaments:	Superior glenohumeral ligament
	Middle glenohumeral ligament
	Inferior glenohumeral ligament
	Coracohumeral ligament
	Coracoacromial ligament
Joint orientation:	Glenoid: Lateral, ventral, caudal
	Humerus: Medial, dorsal, cranial
Type of joint:	Synovial
Articular surface anatomy:	Ovoid
	Glenoid: Concave
	Humerus: Convex
Resting position:	55 to 70 degrees of abduction, 30 degrees of horizontal adduction, neutral rotation
Close-packed position:	Maximal abduction and external rotation
Capsular pattern of restriction:	External rotation > abduction > internal rotation

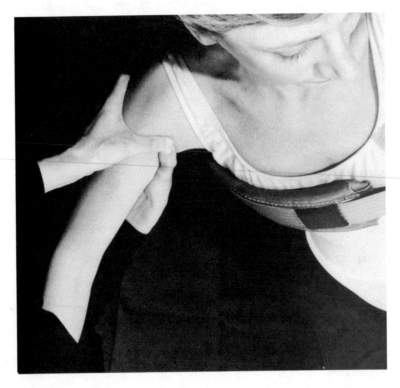

Distraction: (Fig 2–2)

Purpose

- To increase joint play in the glenohumeral joint
- To increase overall range of motion in the glenohumeral joint
- To decrease pain in the glenohumeral joint
- To increase nutrition to articular structures

Positioning

1. The patient is supine.
2. The glenohumeral joint is positioned in the resting position if conservative techniques are indicated, or approximating the restricted range if more aggressive techniques are indicated.
3. A belt should be used to hold the patient's scapula against the trunk, especially in the presence of scapulothoracic hypermobility or increased movement at the scapulothoracic joint with shoulder elevation.
4. The clinician is at the patient's side facing the glenohumeral joint.
5. Both hands grip the proximal humerus from the medial and lateral sides.
6. The clinician can support the patient's forearm and hand by positioning them between the clinician's upper arm and trunk.

Procedure

1. Both hands move the humeral head away from the glenoid joint surface at a 90-degree angle, thus imparting a lateral, ventral, and caudal force to the glenohumeral joint.

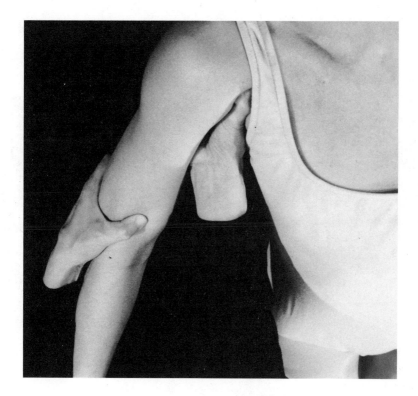

Caudal Glide: First Technique (Fig 2–3)

Purpose

- To increase joint play in the glenohumeral joint
- To increase range of motion into glenohumeral abduction
- To decrease pain in the glenohumeral joint
- To increase nutrition to articular structures

Positioning

1. The patient is supine.
2. The glenohumeral joint is positioned as closely to full adduction as possible.
3. The clinician is positioned between the patient's arm and trunk, facing away from the patient.
4. The clinician can support the patient's forearm and hand by positioning them between the clinician's upper arm and trunk.
5. The stabilizing hand is positioned in the axilla.
6. The manipulating hand grips the distal humerus.

Procedure

1. The stabilizing hand holds the scapula in position against the trunk.
2. The manipulating hand glides the humerus caudally as the clinician rotates his or her trunk away from the joint.

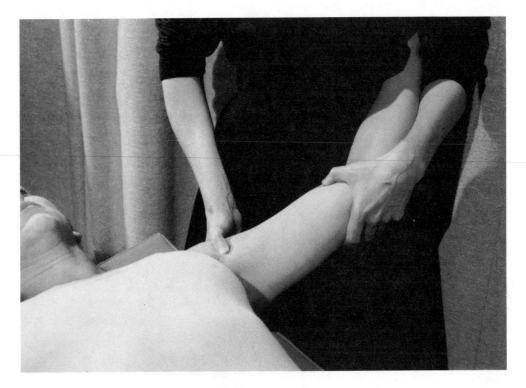

Caudal Glide: Second Technique (Fig 2–4)

Purpose

- To increase joint play in the glenohumeral joint
- To increase range of motion into glenohumeral abduction
- To decrease pain in the glenohumeral joint
- To increase nutrition to articular structures

Positioning

1. The patient is supine.
2. The glenohumeral joint is positioned in the resting position if conservative techniques are indicated, or approximating the restricted range if more aggressive techniques are indicated.
3. A belt can be used to hold the patient's scapula against the trunk.
4. The clinician is at the patient's head facing the glenohumeral joint.
5. The clinician can support the patient's forearm and hand by positioning them between the clinician's upper arm and trunk.
6. The manipulating hand is positioned with the web space over the cranial surface of the proximal humerus.
7. The guiding hand supports the upper limb from the medial side of the distal humerus.

Procedure:

1. The manipulating hand glides the humerus in a caudal direction.
2. The guiding hand controls the position of the humerus.

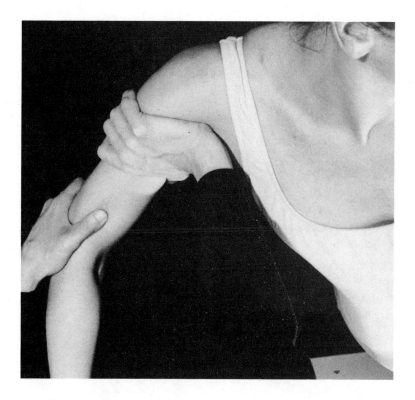

Dorsal Glide (Fig 2–5)

Purpose

- To increase joint play in the glenohumeral joint
- To increase range of motion into glenohumeral internal rotation
- To increase range of motion into glenohumeral flexion
- To increase range of motion into glenohumeral horizontal adduction
- To decrease pain in the glenohumeral joint
- To increase nutrition to articular structures

Positioning

1. The patient is supine with the glenohumeral joint positioned off the edge of the table.
2. The glenohumeral joint is positioned in the resting position if conservative techniques are indicated or approximating the restricted range if more aggressive techniques are indicated.
3. A belt can be used to hold the patient's scapula against the trunk.
4. The clinician is positioned between the patient's arm and trunk, facing away from the patient.
5. The clinician can support the patient's forearm and hand by positioning them between the clinician's upper arm and trunk.
6. The manipulating hand is positioned over the ventral surface of the proximal humerus.
7. The guiding hand supports the upper limb from the dorsal side of the distal humerus.

Procedure (Fig 2—6)

1. The manipulating hand glides the humerus in a dorsal direction.
2. The guiding hand controls the position of the humerus.
3. When approximating the restricted range for horizontal adduction, the dorsal glide can be directed through the shaft of the humerus if the shoulder joint can be positioned in at least 90 degrees of horizontal adduction, as shown below.

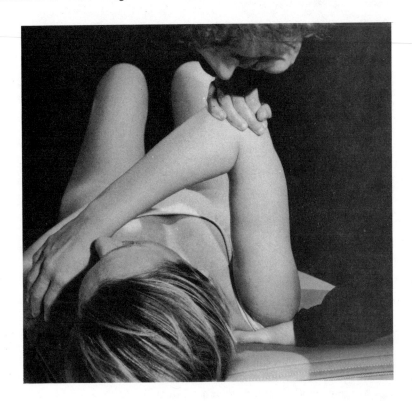

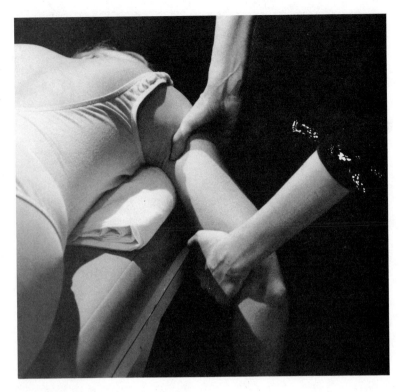

Ventral Glide: First Technique (Fig 2–7)

Purpose

- To increase joint play in the glenohumeral joint
- To increase range of motion into glenohumeral external rotation
- To increase range of motion into glenohumeral extension
- To increase range of motion into glenohumeral horizontal abduction
- To decrease pain in the glenohumeral joint
- To increase nutrition to articular structures

Positioning

1. The patient is prone with the humerus positioned off the edge of the table and a pillow supporting the coracoid process.
2. The glenohumeral joint is positioned in the resting position if conservative techniques are indicated or approximating the restricted range if more aggressive techniques are indicated.
3. A belt can be used to hold the patient's scapula against the trunk.
4. The clinician is at the patient's side facing the glenohumeral joint.
5. The manipulating hand is positioned over the dorsal surface of the proximal humerus.
6. The guiding hand supports the upper limb from the ventral side of the distal humerus.

Procedure

1. The manipulating hand glides the humerus in a ventral direction.
2. The guiding hand controls the position of the humerus.

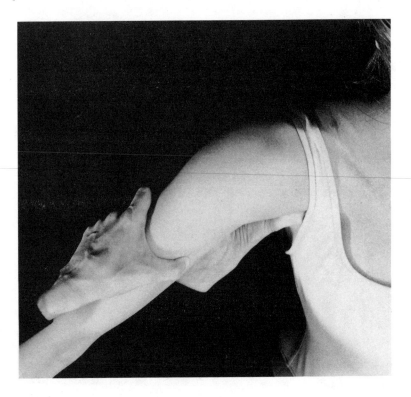

Ventral Glide: Second Technique (Fig 2–8)

Purpose

- To increase joint play in the glenohumeral joint
- To increase range of motion into glenohumeral external rotation
- To increase range of motion into glenohumeral extension
- To increase range of motion into glenohumeral horizontal abduction
- To decrease pain in the glenohumeral joint
- To increase nutrition to articular structures

Positioning

1. The patient is supine.
2. The glenohumeral joint positioned in the resting position if conservative techniques are indicated or approximating the restricted range if more aggressive techniques are indicated.
3. A belt can be used to hold the patient's scapula against the trunk.
4. The clinician is at the patient's side facing the glenohumeral joint.
5. The clinician can support the patient's forearm and hand by positioning them between the clinician's upper arm and trunk.
6. The manipulating hand is positioned over the dorsal surface of the proximal humerus.
7. The guiding hand supports the upper limb from the ventral side of the distal humerus.

Procedure

1. The manipulating hand glides the humerus in a ventral direction.
2. The guiding hand controls the position of the humerus.

Sternoclavicular Joint

Osteokinematic degrees of freedom:	3 motions:
	   Elevation/depression
	   Protraction/retraction
	   Rotation

Ligaments:	Costoclavicular ligament Interclavicular ligament Posterior sternoclavicular ligament Anterior sternoclavicular ligament
Joint orientation:	Manubrium: Lateral, superior Clavicle: Medial, inferior
Type of joint:	Synovial

Articular surface anatomy:	Sellar
	Manubrium:
	   Concave cranial to caudal (elevation/depression)
	   Convex ventral to dorsal (protraction/retraction)
	Clavicle:
	   Convex cranial to caudal (elevation/depression)
	   Concave ventral to dorsal (protraction/retraction)

Resting position:	Clavicle horizontal, scapula 5 cm lateral to the spinous processes with the superior angle at the second rib and the inferior angle at the seventh rib (i.e., arm at side)
Close: packed position:	Arm maximally elevated
Capsular pattern of restriction:	Full elevation is limited

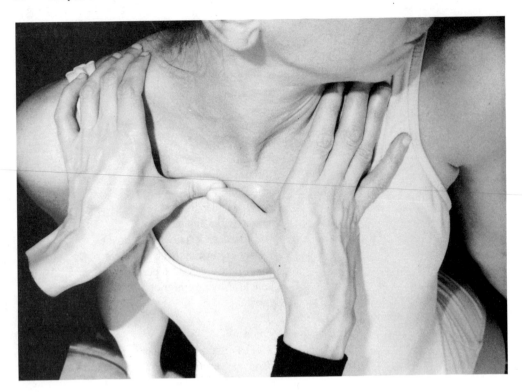

Cranial Glide (Fig 2—9)

(Note head should be positioned forward. Was positioned in rotation to better visualize the joint.)

Purpose

- To increase joint play in the sternoclavicular joint
- To increase range of motion into shoulder depression
- To decrease pain in the sternoclavicular joint
- To increase nutrition to articular structures

Positioning

1. The patient is supine.
2. The joint is in the resting position.
3. The clinician is at the patient's side facing the sternoclavicular joint.
4. The manipulating hand is positioned with the thumb over the thumb of the guiding hand.
5. The guiding hand is positioned with the thumb over the caudal surface of the clavicle about 3 cm lateral to the most medial aspect.

Procedure

1. The manipulating hand glides the clavicle in a cranial direction.
2. The guiding hand controls the position of the manipulating hand.

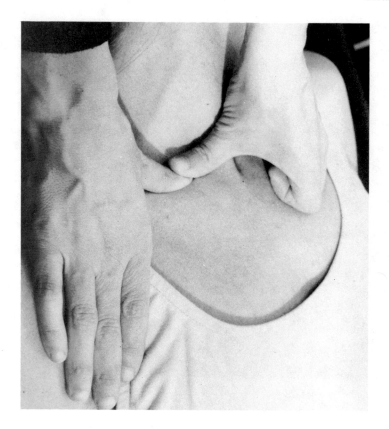

Caudal Glide (Fig 2–10)

Purpose

- To increase joint play in the sternoclavicular joint
- To increase range of motion into shoulder elevation
- To decrease pain in the sternoclavicular joint
- To increase nutrition to articular structures

Positioning

1. The patient is supine.
2. The joint is in the resting position.
3. The clinician is at the patient's head facing the sternoclavicular joint.
4. The manipulating hand is positioned with the thumb over the thumb of the guiding hand.
5. The guiding hand is positioned with the thumb over the cranial surface of the clavicle about 3 cm lateral to the most medial aspect.

Procedure

1. The manipulating hand glides the clavicle in a caudal direction.
2. The guiding hand controls the position of the manipulating hand.

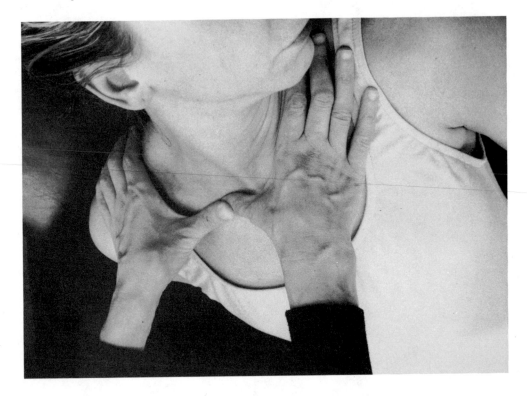

Dorsal Glide (Fig 2–11)

(Note head should be positioned forward. Was positioned in rotation to better visualize the joint.)

Purpose

- To increase joint play in the sternoclavicular joint
- To increase range of motion into shoulder retraction
- To decrease pain in the sternoclavicular joint
- To increase nutrition to articular structures

Positioning

1. The patient is supine.
2. The joint is in the resting position.
3. The clinician is at the patient's side facing the sternoclavicular joint.
4. The manipulating hand is positioned with the thumb over the thumb of the guiding hand.
5. The guiding hand is positioned with the thumb over the ventral surface of the clavicle about 3 cm lateral to the most medial aspect.

Procedure

1. The manipulating hand glides the clavicle in a dorsal direction.
2. The guiding hand controls the position of the manipulating hand.

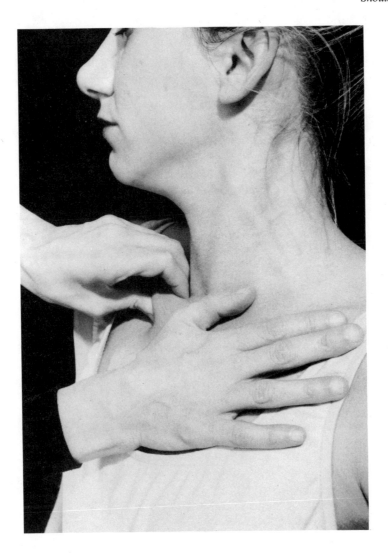

Ventral Glide (Fig 2–12)

Purpose

- To increase joint play in the sternoclavicular joint
- To increase range of motion into shoulder protraction
- To decrease pain in the sternoclavicular joint
- To increase nutrition to articular structures

Positioning

1. The patient is supine.
2. The joint is in the resting position.
3. The clinician is at the patient's side facing the patient's sternoclavicular joint.
4. The stabilizing hand is positioned over the patient's sternum.
5. The manipulation hand grips around the clavicle to the ventral surface with the fingers.

Procedure

1. The stabilizing hand holds the sternum in position.
2. The manipulating hand glides the clavicle in a ventral direction.

Acromioclavicular Joint

Osteokinematic degrees of freedom:	3 motions:
	  Elevation/depression
	  Protraction/retraction
	  Rotation

Ligaments:	Superior acromioclavicular ligament Inferior acromioclavicular ligament Coracoclavicular ligaments (conoid and trapezoid)
Joint orientation:	Acromion: Cranial, medial, ventral Clavicle: Caudal, lateral, dorsal
Type of joint:	Synovial
Joint surface anatomy:	Ovoid Acromion: Concave Clavicle: Convex
Resting position:	Clavicle horizontal, scapula 5 cm lateral to the spinous processes with the superior angle at the second rib and the inferior angle at the seventh rib (i.e., arm at side)
Close-packed position:	Arm abducted 90 degrees
Capsular pattern of restriction:	Full elevation is limited

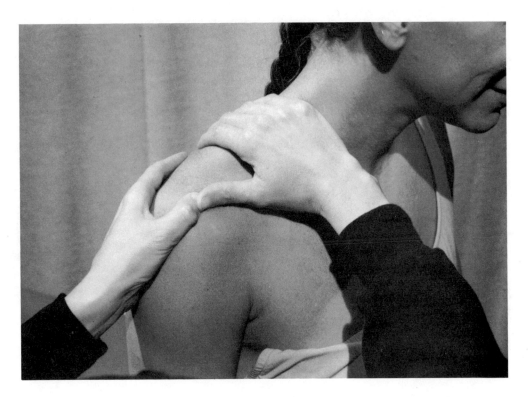

Dorsal Glide (Fig 2–13)

Purpose

- To increase joint play in the acromioclavicular joint
- To increase range of motion into shoulder elevation
- To decrease pain in the acromioclavicular joint
- To increase nutrition to articular structures

Positioning

1. The patient is sitting.
2. The joint is in the resting position.
3. The clinician is facing the ventral surface of the acromioclavicular joint.
4. The stabilizing hand is positioned over the dorsal surface of the scapula.
5. The manipulating hand is positioned with the thumb over the thumb of the guiding hand.
6. The guiding hand, which is the same hand as the stabilizing hand, is positioned with the thumb over the ventrolateral surface of the clavicle.

Procedure

1. The stabilizing hand holds the scapula in position.
2. The manipulating hand glides the clavicle in a dorsal direction.
3. The guiding hand controls the position of the manipulating hand.

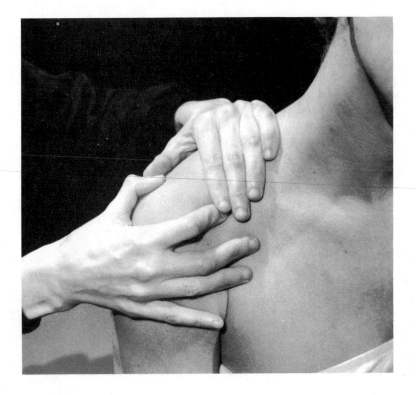

Ventral Glide (Fig 2–14)

Purpose

- To increase joint play in the acromioclavicular joint
- To increase range of motion into shoulder elevation
- To decrease pain in the acromioclavicular joint
- To increase nutrition to articular structures

Positioning

1. The patient is sitting.
2. The joint is in the resting position.
3. The clinician is facing the dorsal surface of the acromioclavicular joint.
4. The stabilizing hand is positioned over the acromion and over the ventral surface of the proximal humerus.
5. The manipulating hand is positioned with the thumb over the thumb of the guiding hand.
6. The guiding hand, which is the same hand as the stabilizing hand, is positioned over the dorsolateral surface of the clavicle.

Procedure

1. The stabilizing hand holds the acromion in position.
2. The manipulating hand glides the clavicle in a ventral direction.
3. The guiding hand controls the position of the manipulating hand.

Scapulothoracic Joint

Osteokinematic degrees of freedom:	3 motions:
	Protraction/retraction
	Elevation/depression (accompanied by rotation)
	Scapular winging
Ligaments:	None
Joint orientation:	Thorax: Dorsal, lateral, cranial
	Scapula: Ventral, medial, caudal
Type of joint:	Functional articulation
Joint surface anatomy:	Ovoid
	Thorax: Convex
	Scapula: Concave
Resting position:	Clavicle horizontal, scapula 5 cm lateral to the spinous processes with the superior angle at the second rib and the inferior angle at the seventh rib (i.e., arm at side)
Close-packed position:	None; not a synovial joint
Capsular pattern of restriction:	None; not a synovial joint

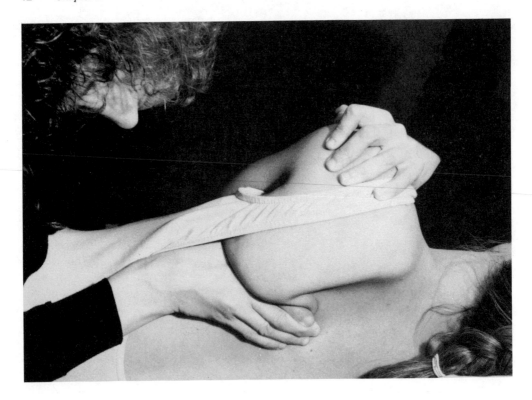

Distraction (Fig 2–15)

Purpose

- To increase joint play in the scapulothoracic joint
- To increase overall range of motion in the scapulothoracic joint
- To increase range of motion into scapular winging
- To decrease pain in the scapulothoracic joint

Positioning

1. The patient is lying on his or her side with the arm supported on a pillow or on the clinician's arm.
2. The joint is in the resting position.
3. The clinician is facing the patient's shoulder.
4. The manipulating hand is positioned over the acromion.
5. The guiding hand is positioned adjacent to the inferior angle of the scapula.

Procedure

1. The manipulating hand moves the scapula medially and caudally over the guiding hand.
2. The guiding hand lifts the scapula away from the ribs.

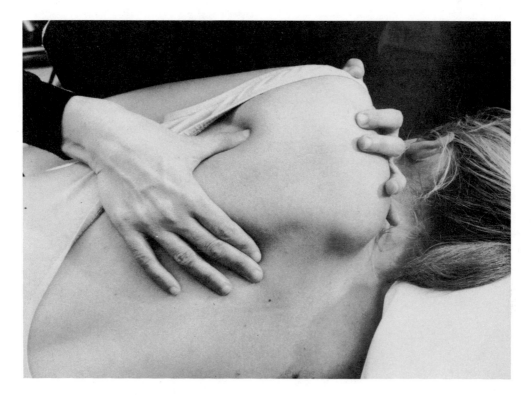

Cranial Glide (Fig 2–16)

Purpose

- To increase joint play in the scapulothoracic joint
- To increase range of motion into scapular elevation
- To increase range of motion into scapular lateral rotation
- To decrease pain in the scapulothoracic joint

Positioning

1. The patient is side-lying with the arm supported on a pillow or on the clinician's arm.
2. The joint is in the resting position.
3. The clinician is facing the patient's shoulder.
4. The manipulating hand is positioned over the inferior angle of the scapula.
5. The guiding hand is positioned over the acromion.

Procedure

1. The manipulating hand glides the scapula in a cranial direction.
2. The guiding hand controls the position of the scapula.

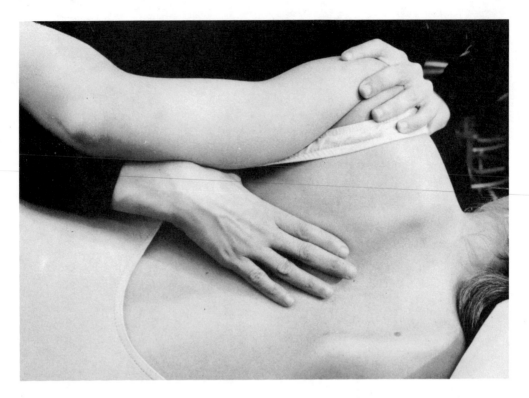

Caudal Glide (Fig 2–17)

Purpose

- To increase joint play in the scapulothoracic joint
- To increase range of motion into scapular depression
- To increase range of motion into scapular medial rotation
- To decrease pain in the scapulothoracic joint

Positioning

1. The patient is side-lying with the arm supported on a pillow or on the clinician's arm.
2. The joint is in the resting position.
3. The clinician is facing the patient's shoulder.
4. The manipulating hand is positioned over the acromion.
5. The guiding hand is positioned over the inferior angle of the scapula.

Procedure

1. The manipulating hand glides the acromion in a caudal direction.
2. The guiding hand controls the position of the scapula.

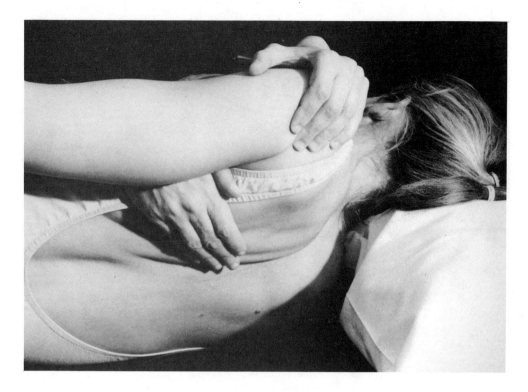

Medial Glide (Fig 2–18)

Purpose

- To increase joint play in the scapulothoracic joint
- To increase range of motion into scapular retraction
- To increase range of motion into scapular depression
- To increase range of motion into scapular medial rotation
- To decrease pain in the scapulothoracic joint

Positioning

1. The patient is side-lying with the arm supported on a pillow or on the clinician's arm.
2. The joint is in the resting position.
3. The clinician is facing the patient's shoulder.
4. Both hands are positioned over the lateral surface of the scapula, one hand over the axillary border and the other hand over the acromion.

Procedure

1. Both hands glide the scapula in a medial direction.

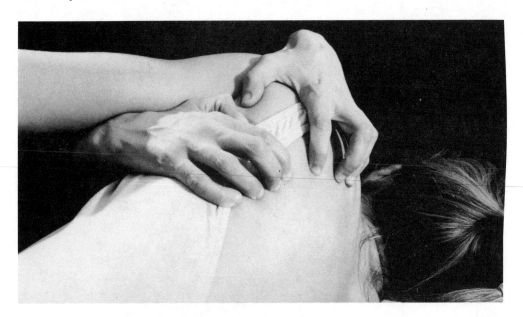

Lateral Glide (Fig 2–19)

Purpose

- To increase joint play in the scapulothoracic joint
- To increase range of motion into scapular protraction
- To increase range of motion into scapular elevation
- To increase range of motion into scapular lateral rotation
- To decrease pain in the scapulothoracic joint

Positioning

1. The patient is side-lying with the arm supported on a pillow or on the clinician's arm.
2. The joint is in the resting position.
3. The clinician is facing the patient's shoulder.
4. Both hands are positioned with the fingertips over the vertebral border of the scapula.

Procedure

1. Both hands glide the scapula in a lateral direction.

REFERENCES

1. Bagg SD, Forrest WJ: A biomechanical analysis of scapular rotation during arm abduction in the scapular plane. *Am J Phys Med Rehabil* 1988; 67:238.
2. Blakely RL, Palmer ML: Analysis of rotation accompanying shoulder flexion. *Phys Ther* 1984; 64:1214.
3. Freedman L, Munro RR: Abduction of the arm in the scapular plane: Scapular and glenohumeral movements. *J Bone Joint Surg [Br]* 1966; 48A:1503.
4. Hart DL, Carmichael SW: Biomechanics of the shoulder. *Phys Ther* 1985; 6:229.
5. Hertling D, Kessler RM: The shoulder and shoulder girdle, in Hertling D, Kessler RM: *Management of Common Musculoskeletal Disorders,* ed 2. Philadelphia, JB Lippincott, 1990.
6. Palmer ML, Blakely RL: Documentation of medial rotation accompanying shoulder flexion. *Phys Ther* 1986; 66:55.
7. Peat M: Functional anatomy of the shoulder complex. *Phys Ther* 1986; 66:1855.
8. Peat M: The shoulder complex: A review of some aspects of functional anatomy. *Physiotherapy Canada* 1977; 29:241.
9. Rothman RH, Marvel JP, Heppenstall RB: Anatomic considerations in the glenohumeral joint. *Orthop Clin North Am* 1975; 6:341.
10. Sarrafian SK: Gross and functional anatomy of the shoulder. *Clin Orthop* 1983; 173:11.
11. Turkel SJ et al: Stabilizing mechanisms preventing anterior dislocation of the glenohumeral joint. *J Bone Joint Surg* 1981; 63A:1208.

Figure **3 – 1**

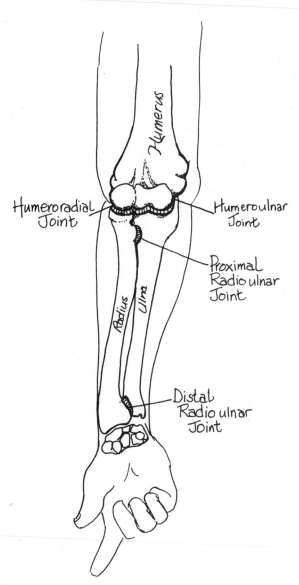

Elbow and Forearm Joints

Chapter 3

Elbow and Forearm

The elbow joint generally is classified as a hinge joint.[3] Flexion and extension occur at the humeroulnar and humeroradial joints. Pronation and supination are considered motions of the forearm and take place at the humeroradial, proximal radioulnar, distal radioulnar, and ulnomeniscotriquetral joints. Most functional activities occur between 30 and 130 degrees of flexion, and between 50 degrees of pronation and 50 degrees of supination.[6]

Positional faults are not uncommon at the humeroradial joint. Proximal positional faults frequently occur after a fall on an outstretched arm. Distal positional faults often result from a pull on the patient's arm, and therefore are especially common in young children.

FLEXION AND EXTENSION

Medial and lateral gapping and gliding are the primary oscillation techniques used to restore extension and flexion at the humeroulnar joint. Dorsal and ventral glides, which ordinarily would be the appropriate techniques for restoring these motions, are ineffective, because the ulnar articular surface encompasses such a large arc in the frontal plane that the two joint surfaces jam together when these manipulation techniques are attempted. Therefore the only approaches available to increase joint play at the humeroulnar joint are medial and lateral techniques and distraction. This does not hold true for the humeroradial joint. Since it is a shallow joint consisting of a convex humerus and a concave radius, dorsal and ventral glides are effective in restoring extension and flexion, respectively.

Distraction techniques for all joints are performed so that the bone being manipulated is guided perpendicular to the treatment plane. Because the proximal ulna is angulated 45 degrees ventral to the shaft of the ulna, and thus the shaft of the ulna is not perpendicular to the treatment plane, humeroulnar distraction manipulation must occur at a 45-degree angle from the position of the shaft of the ulna (see Fig 1–4,A and B).

Flexion is accompanied by adduction or varus angulation at the elbow, and extension by abduction or valgus angulation. This occurs in part because the medial trochlear surface of the humerus is more distal than the capitulum[1, 5, 7] and in part because the medial joint surfaces gap with extension and the lateral joint surfaces gap with flexion.[7] Emphasizing medial gapping when treating to restore extension and lateral gapping when treating to restore flexion thus will produce gains in range of motion.

The anterior fibers of the medial collateral ligament are the primary stabilizers of the elbow.[2, 4, 8, 9] This stabilization most likely occurs throughout the range of motion.[2, 4, 9] Restoring normal mobility in this ligament with medial gapping techniques therefore is especially important when increasing range of motion into both flexion and extension.

PRONATION AND SUPINATION

Most motion into pronation and supination occurs simultaneously at the proximal and distal radioulnar joints. The ulnomeniscotriquetral joint contributes a small amount to pronation and supination at the end of range (see Chapter 4 for manipulation techniques). When the ulna is stationary the radius rotates ventrally and medially with pronation,[7] and dorsally and laterally with supination. Pronation is accompanied by a dorsal glide of the radius on the ulna proximally and a ventral glide of the radius on the ulna distally; the reverse occurs with supination. Restoring motion into pronation and supination, respectively, thus entails gliding in the aforementioned directions. Because the medial collateral ligament also checks pronation,[9] normalizing the kinematics for medial gapping also will improve range into pronation. The radius also spins on the humerus during pronation and supination. Although there is no technique to restore spinning directly, normalizing the kinematics at the humeroradial joint using all available joint manipulation techniques and performing passive range of motion into pronation and supination will aid significantly in the restoration of the spinning motion.

Humeroulnar Joint

Osteokinematic degrees of freedom:	2 motions: Flexion/extension Abduction/adduction
Ligaments:	Ulnar collateral ligament
Joint orientation:	Humerus: caudal, dorsal; note, however, that the trochlear notch forms a 45-degree angle with the shaft of the ulna Ulna: cranial, ventral
Type of joint:	Synovial
Articular surface anatomy:	Sellar: Humerous Concave medial to lateral (abduction/adduction) Convex ventral to dorsal (flexion/extension) Ulna: Convex medial to lateral (abduction/adduction) Concave ventral to dorsal (flexion/extension)
Resting position:	70 degrees flexion, 10 degrees supination
Close-packed position:	Full extension and supination
Capsular pattern of restriction:	Flexion > extension Pronation and supination are limited only if condition is severe

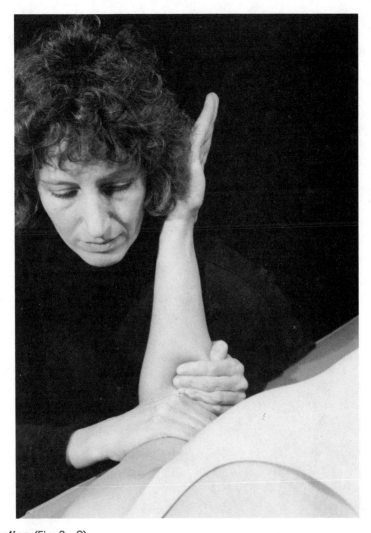

Distraction (Fig 3-2)

Purpose

- To increase joint play in the humeroulnar joint
- To increase overall range of motion in the elbow joint
- To decrease pain in the elbow
- To increase nutrition to articular structures

Positioning

1. The patient is sitting or supine.
2. The humeroulnar joint is positioned in the resting position if conservative techniques are indicated or approximating the restricted range if more aggressive techniques are indicated.
3. The clinician is at the patient's hip, facing the humeroulnar joint, with the patient's upper arm resting on the table and the distal forearm resting on the clinician's shoulder.
4. The stabilizing hand grips the distal humerus from the ventral side.

5. Instead of or in addition to the stabilizing hand, a belt can be used to hold the patient's humerus to the table.
6. The manipulating hand grips the proximal ulna from the ventral side.

Procedure

1. The stabilizing hand holds the distal humerus against the table.
2. The manipulating hand moves the proximal ulna away from the humeral joint surface at a 90-degree angle from the treatment plane, or at an angle that is in 45 degrees less flexion than the position of the ulnar shaft.

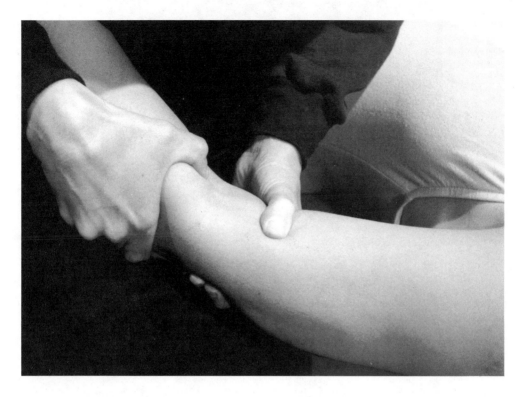

Medial Glide (Fig 3–3)

Purpose

- To increase joint play in the humeroulnar joint
- To increase range of motion into elbow abduction
- To increase range of motion into elbow extension
- To increase range of motion into elbow flexion
- To decrease pain in the elbow
- To increase nutrition to articular structures

Positioning

1. The patient is sitting or supine.
2. The humeroulnar joint is positioned in the resting position if conservative techniques are indicated or approximating the restricted range if more aggressive techniques are indicated.
3. The clinician is facing the patient between the patient's arm and trunk with the patient's forearm between the clinician's upper arm and trunk.
4. The stabilizing hand grips the distal humerus from the medial side.
5. The manipulating hand grips the proximal radius from the lateral side.

Procedure

1. The stabilizing hand holds the humerus in position.
2. The manipulating hand glides the proximal ulna in a medial direction indirectly through the radius while the therapist's trunk guides the motion.

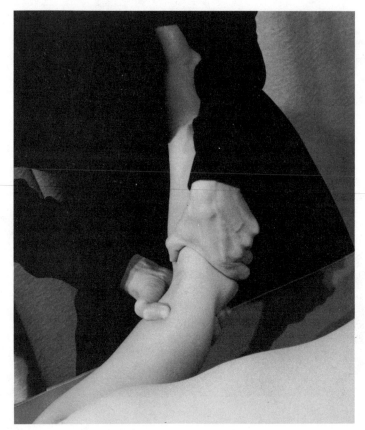

Lateral Glide (Fig 3–4)

Purpose

- To increase joint play in the humeroulnar joint
- To increase range of motion into elbow adduction
- To increase range of motion into elbow extension
- To increase range of motion into elbow flexion
- To decrease pain in the elbow
- To increase nutrition to articular structures

Positioning

1. The patient is sitting or supine.
2. The humeroulnar joint is positioned in the resting position if conservative techniques are indicated or approximating the restricted range if more aggressive techniques are indicated.
3. The clinician is at the patient's side facing the humeroulnar joint with the patient's forearm between the clinician's upper arm and trunk.
4. The stabilizing hand grips the distal humerus from the lateral side.
5. The manipulating hand grips the proximal ulna from the medial side.

Procedure

1. The stabilizing hand holds the humerus in position.
2. The manipulating hand glides the proximal ulna in a lateral direction while the therapist's trunk guides the motion.

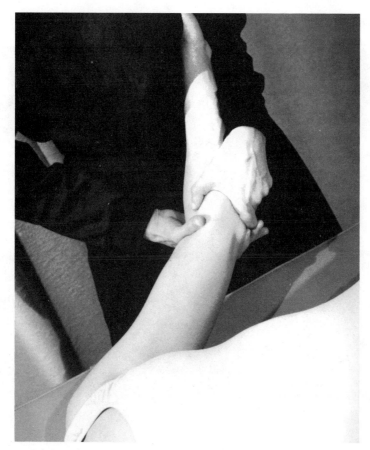

Medial Gap (Fig 3-5)

Purpose

- To increase joint play in the humeroulnar joint
- To increase range of motion into elbow extension
- To increase range of motion into elbow flexion
- To increase range of motion into forearm pronation
- To decrease pain in the elbow
- To increase nutrition to articular structures

Positioning

1. The patient is sitting or supine.
2. The humeroulnar joint is positioned in slight flexion.
3. The clinician is at the patient's side, facing the humeroulnar joint with the patient's forearm between the clinician's upper arm and trunk.
4. The stabilizing hand supports the forearm from the ulnar side and holds it against the clinician's trunk.
5. The manipulating hand grips the lateral side of the elbow at the joint line.

Procedure

1. The stabilizing hand holds the forearm in position.
2. The manipulating hand moves the elbow at the lateral joint line in a medial direction, thus creating a gapping at the joint line medially.

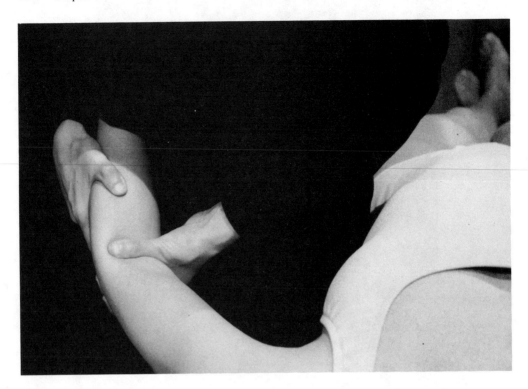

Lateral Gap (Fig 3–6)

Purpose

- To increase joint play in the humeroulnar joint
- To increase range of motion into elbow flexion
- To decrease pain in the elbow
- To increase nutrition to articular structures

Positioning

1. The patient is sitting or supine.
2. The humeroulnar joint is positioned in slight flexion.
3. The clinician is facing the patient between the patient's arm and trunk with the patient's forearm between the clinician's upper arm and trunk.
4. The stabilizing hand supports the forearm from the radial side and holds it against the clinician's trunk.
5. The manipulating hand grips the medial side of the elbow at the joint line.

Procedure

1. The stabilizing hand holds the forearm in position.
2. The manipulating hand moves the elbow at the medial joint line in a lateral direction, thus creating a gapping at the joint line laterally.

Humeroradial Joint

Osteokinematic degrees of freedom:	3 motions: Flexion/extension Pronation/supination Abduction/adduction
Ligaments:	Radial collateral ligament
Joint orientation:	Humerus: Caudal Radius: Cranial
Type of joint:	Synovial
Articular surface anatomy:	Ovoid Humerus: Convex Radius: Concave
Resting position:	Full extension and supination
Close-packed position:	90 degrees flexion, 5 degrees supination
Capsular pattern of restriction:	Flexion > extension Pronation and supination are limited only if condition is severe

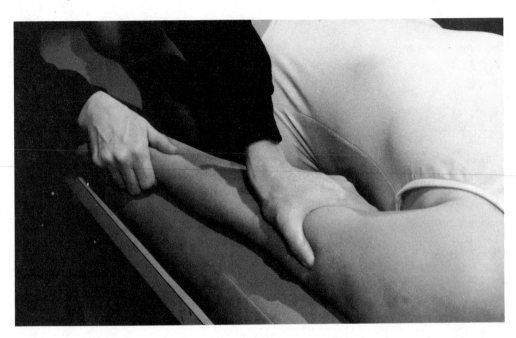

Distraction (Fig 3–7)

Purpose

- To increase joint play in the humeroradial joint
- To increase overall range of motion in the humeroradial joint
- To reduce a proximal positional fault
- To decrease pain at the elbow
- To increase nutrition to articular structures

Positioning

1. The patient is sitting or supine.
2. The humeroradial joint is positioned in the resting position if conservative techniques are indicated for stretching or pain reduction or if a positional fault is being treated, or approximating the restricted range if more aggressive techniques are indicated for stretching or pain reduction.
3. The clinician is between the patient's arm and trunk facing the humeroradial joint.
4. The stabilizing hand grips the distal humerus from the ventral side.
5. The manipulating hand grips the distal radius.

Procedure

1. The stabilizing hand holds the humerus in position.
2. The manipulating hand moves the radial head distally.

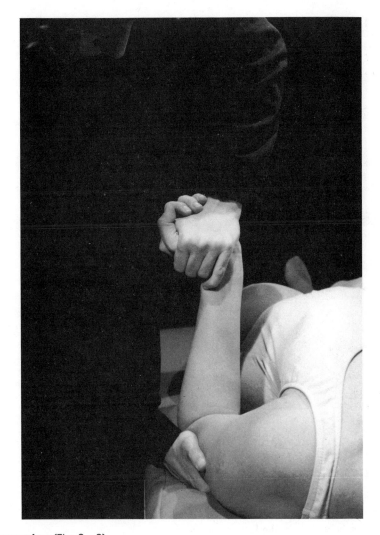

Compression (Fig 3–8)

Purpose

- To reduce a distal positional fault of the radius

Positioning

1. The patient is sitting or supine.
2. The elbow joint is positioned in 90 degrees of flexion, and the wrist is extended.
3. The clinician is at the patient's side facing the humeroradial joint.
4. The stabilizing hand grips the distal humerus from the dorsal side.
5. The manipulating hand grips the patient's hand on the volar surface.

Procedure

1. The stabilizing hand holds the humerus in position.
2. The manipulating hand moves the shaft of the radius downward indirectly through the wrist.

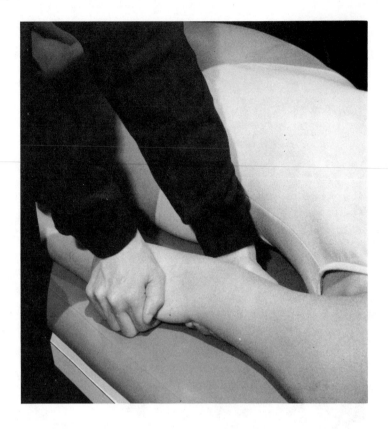

Dorsal Glide (Fig 3–9)

Purpose

- To increase joint play in the humeroradial joint
- To increase range of motion into elbow extension
- To decrease pain in the elbow
- To increase nutrition to articular structures

Positioning

1. The patient is sitting or supine.
2. The humeroradial joint is positioned in the resting position if conservative techniques are indicated or approximating the restricted range if more aggressive techniques are indicated.
3. The clinician is at the patient's side facing the humeroradial joint.
4. The stabilizing hand grips the distal humerus from the dorsal side.
5. The manipulating hand grips the proximal radius from the ventral side.

Procedure

1. The stabilizing hand holds the humerus in position.
2. The manipulating hand glides the proximal radius in a dorsal direction.

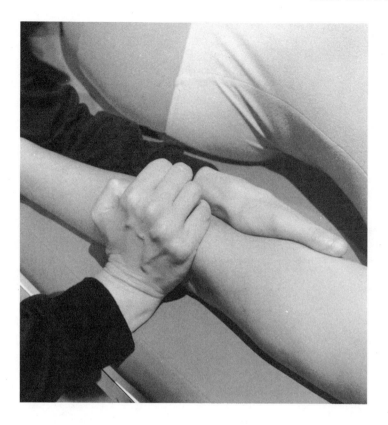

Ventral Glide (Fig 3-10)

Purpose

- To increase joint play in the humeroradial joint
- To increase range of motion into elbow flexion
- To decrease pain in the elbow
- To increase nutrition to articular structures

Positioning

1. The patient is sitting or supine.
2. The humeroradial joint is positioned in the resting position if conservative techniques are indicated, or approximating the restricted range if more aggressive techniques are indicated.
3. The clinician is at the patient's side facing the humeroradial joint.
4. The stabilizing hand grips the distal humerus from the ventral side.
5. The manipulating hand grips the proximal radius from the dorsal side.

Procedure

1. The stabilizing hand holds the humerus in position.
2. The manipulating hand glides the proximal radius in a ventral direction.

Proximal Radioulnar Joint

Osteokinematic degrees of freedom:	1 motion: Pronation/supination
Ligaments:	Annular ligament Quadrate ligament Interosseous membrane
Joint orientation:	Ulna: Lateral, ventral Radius: Medial, dorsal
Type of joint:	Synovial
Articular surface anatomy:	Ovoid Ulna: Concave Radius: Convex
Resting position:	35 degrees supination, 70 degrees flexion
Close-packed position:	5 degrees supination, full extension
Capsular pattern of restriction:	Supination = pronation

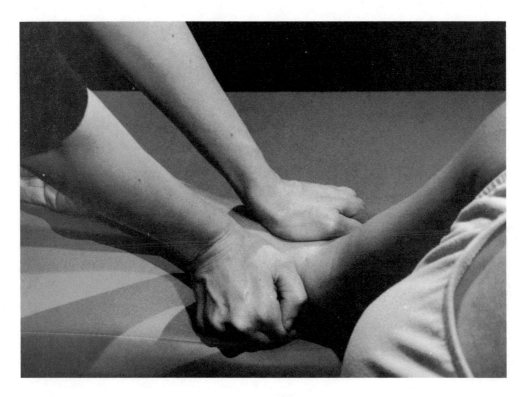

Dorsal Glide of Radial Head (Fig 3–11)

Purpose

- To increase joint play in the proximal radioulnar joint
- To increase range of motion into forearm pronation
- To decrease pain in the elbow
- To increase nutrition to articular structures

Positioning

1. The patient is sitting.
2. The proximal radioulnar joint is positioned in the resting position if conservative techniques are indicated or approximating the restricted range if more aggressive techniques are indicated.
3. The clinician is at the patient's side facing the proximal radioulnar joint.
4. The stabilizing hand grips the proximal ulna from the dorsal side.
5. The manipulating hand grips the radial head ventrally.

Procedure

1. The stabilizing hand holds the ulna in position.
2. The manipulating hand glides the radial head in a dorsal direction.

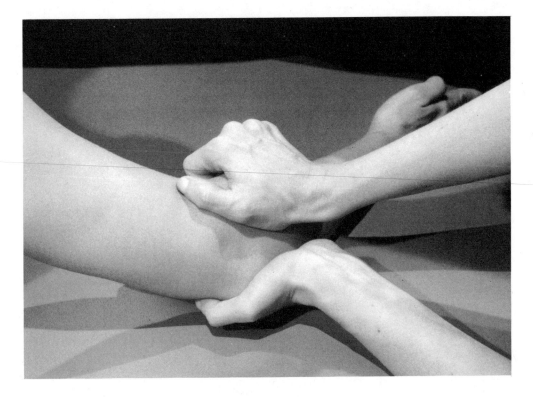

Ventral Glide of Radial Head (Fig 3–12)

Purpose

- To increase joint play in the proximal radioulnar joint
- To increase range of motion into forearm supination
- To decrease pain in the elbow
- To increase nutrition to articular structures

Positioning

1. The patient is sitting.
2. The proximal radioulnar joint is positioned in the resting position if conservative techniques are indicated or approximating the restricted range if more aggressive techniques are indicated.
3. The clinician is at the patient's side facing the proximal radioulnar joint.
4. The stabilizing hand grips the proximal ulna from the ventral side.
5. The manipulating hand grips the radial head dorsally.

Procedure

1. The stabilizing hand holds the ulna in position.
2. The manipulating hand glides the radial head in a ventral direction.

Distal Radioulnar Joint

Osteokinematic degrees of freedom:	1 motion: Pronation/supination
Ligaments:	Anterior radioulnar ligament
	Posterior radioulnar ligament
	Interosseous membrane
Joint orientation:	Ulna: Lateral
	Radius: Medial
Type of joint:	Synovial
Articular surface anatomy:	Ovoid
	Ulna: Convex
	Radius: Concave
Resting position:	10 degrees supination
Close-packed position:	5 degrees supination
Capsular pattern of restriction:	Supination = pronation

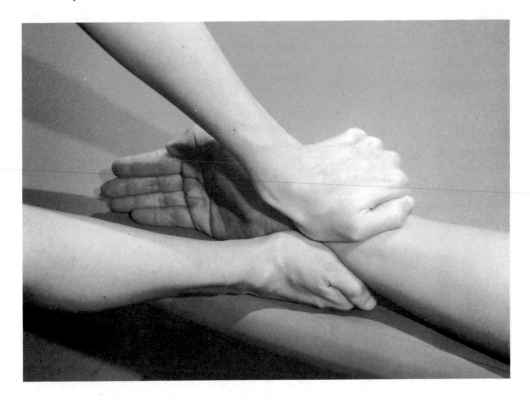

Dorsal Glide of Distal Radius (Fig 3–13)

Purpose

- To increase joint play in the distal radioulnar joint
- To increase range of motion into forearm supination
- To decrease pain in the distal forearm
- To increase nutrition to articular structures

Positioning

1. The patient is sitting.
2. The distal radioulnar joint is positioned in the resting position if conservative techniques are indicated or approximating the restricted range if more aggressive techniques are indicated.
3. The clinician is at the patient's side facing the distal radioulnar joint.
4. The stabilizing hand grips the distal ulna from the dorsal side.
5. The manipulating hand grips the distal radius from the ventral side.

Procedure

1. The stabilizing hand holds the ulna in position.
2. The manipulating hand glides the distal radius in a dorsal direction.

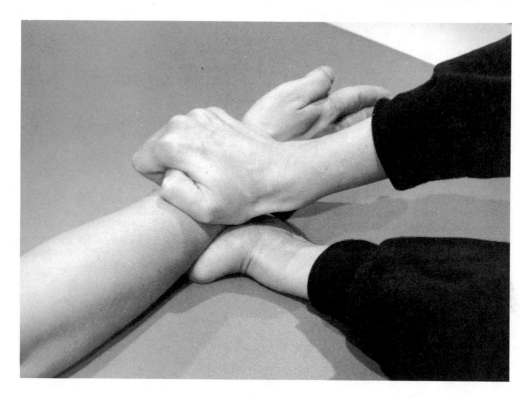

Ventral Glide of Distal Radius (Fig 3–14)

Purpose

- To increase joint play in the distal radioulnar joint
- To increase range of motion into forearm pronation
- To decrease pain in the distal forearm
- To increase nutrition to articular structures

Positioning

1. The patient is sitting.
2. The distal radioulnar joint is positioned in the resting position if conservative techniques are indicated or approximating the restricted range if more aggressive techniques are indicated.
3. The clinician is at the patient's side facing the distal radioulnar joint.
4. The stabilizing hand grips the distal ulna from the ventral side.
5. The manipulating hand grips the distal radius from the dorsal side.

Procedure

1. The stabilizing hand holds the ulna in position.
2. The manipulating hand glides the distal radius in a ventral direction.

REFERENCES

1. Deland JT, Garg A, Walker PS: Biomechanical basis for elbow hinge-distractor design. *Clin Orthop* 1987; 215:303.
2. Hotchkiss RN, Weiland AJ: Valgus stability of the elbow. *J Orthop Res* 1987; 5:372.
3. Ishizuki M: Functional anatomy of the elbow joint and three-dimensional quantitative motion analysis of the elbow joint. *J Jpn Orthop Assoc* 1979; 53:109.
4. Johnson C, Glasheen-Wray MB: Effect of forearm abduction on the ulnar collateral ligament. *Phys Ther* 1983; 63:660.
5. London JT: Kinematics of the elbow. *J Bone Joint Surg [Am]* 1981; 63:529.
6. Morrey BF et al: A biomechanical study of normal functional elbow motion. *J Bone Joint Surg [Am]* 1981; 63:872.
7. Morrey BF, Chao EYS: Passive motion of the elbow joint. *J Bone Joint Surg [Am]* 1976; 58:501.
8. Schwab GH et al: Biomechanics of elbow instability: The role of the medial collateral ligament. *Clin Orthop* 1980; 146:42.
9. Sojbjerg JO, Ovesen J, Nielsen S: Experimental elbow instability after transection of the medial collateral ligament. *Clin Orthop* 1987; 218:186.

Figure **4-1**

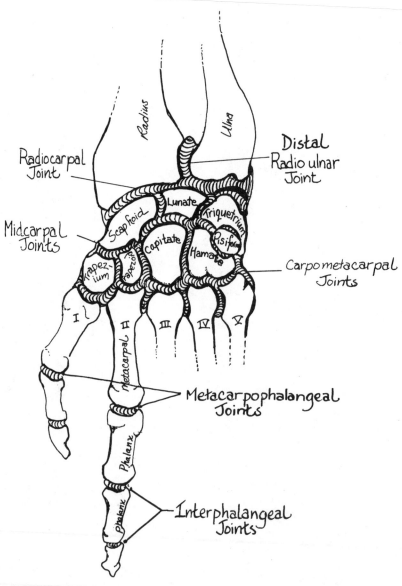

Wrist and Hand Joints

Chapter 4 _____

Wrist and Hand

The wrist is made up of the radiocarpal (radioscaphoid and radiolunate) joint, the ulnocarpal (ulnomeniscotriquetral) joint, the triquetrium-pisiform articulation, and the midcarpal joint. Wrist range of motion is considered functional if 10 degrees of flexion and 35 degrees of extension are present,[1] because this amount of motion allows the wrist to position the hand for skilled activities. The amount of range of motion considered functional for the joints of the hand depends on the task. Motion at the thumb is crucial for hand function because it permits grasp. Most of the mobility at the thumb occurs at the trapeziometacarpal joint, although the metacarpophalangeal and interphalangeal joints of the thumb also contribute to motion. Arching of the hand is an additional component of grasp and occurs at the carpometacarpal and intermetacarpal joints of digits 2 through 5. Finger motion is a product of motion at the second through fifth metacarpophalangeal and interphalangeal joints, and is also a necessary component of grasp.

Positional faults are fairly common in the radiolunate joint, and frequently result from a fall on an outstretched arm.

PRONATION AND SUPINATION

Although the preponderance of the motion for pronation and supination occurs at the humeroradial joint and the proximal and distal radioulnar joints, some motion does occur at the ulnomeniscotriquetral joint. During pronation and supination the disc moves with the triquetrium as it glides across the distal ulnar articulation.[4] Restoring dorsal and ventral motion between the triquetrium and the ulna will produce small range gains into pronation and supination, respectively.

WRIST FLEXION AND EXTENSION

Although there is some evidence that wrist motion is best described as motion occurring among three columns of carpal bones,[3, 5] the most common belief is that wrist motion occurs primarily between the radiocarpal and ulnocarpal row and the midcarpal row.

At the proximal articulation the convex scaphoid, lunate, and triquetrium move on the concave radius and disc. The pisiform articulates on the triquetrium and is not considered a component of the proximal row. Dorsal glides of the scaphoid, lunate, and triquetrium will assist in the restoration of flexion, and volar glide of these bones will help restore extension. Extension is accompanied by supination of the scaphoid, and flexion is accompanied by pronation of the scaphoid.[4] All joint play between the scaphoid and its adjacent carpal bones therefore also must be restored for normal arthrokinematic flexion and extension to occur.

At the midcarpal row the convex distal aspect of the scaphoid moves on the concave trapezium and trapezoid as the concave ulnar aspect of the scaphoid and the lunate and triquetrium move on the convex capitate and hamate.[4] Volar gliding of the trapezium and trapezoid on the scaphoid and dorsal gliding of the capitate and hamate on the scaphoid, lunate, and triquetrium therefore will restore flexion; the opposite holds true for extension. Manipulating the entire distal row of carpal bones on the proximal row is indicated only when both flexion and extension are limited, because volar gliding will restore flexion at the radial articulation and extension at the ulnar articulation, and vice versa for dorsal gliding. Manipulation of individual carpal bones in the appropriate direction is necessary when both flexion and extension range of motion deficits are not being addressed concurrently.

A greater percentage of motion for extension takes place at the radiocarpal and ulnocarpal joints, whereas relatively more motion for flexion occurs at the midcarpal joint.[6, 8, 9] Radiocarpal and ulnocarpal excursion therefore should be emphasized when restoring extension, and midcarpal excursion should be emphasized when restoring flexion.

WRIST RADIAL AND ULNAR DEVIATION

In the frontal plane the proximal row of carpal bones is convex on a concave radius and disc and the distal row is convex on the proximal row of carpals. Restoring ulnar deviation thus entails gliding in a radial direction at both rows, and radial deviation in an ulnar direction at both rows.

Radial deviation occurs in conjunction with flexion, primarily of the scaphoid on the radius[9, 10] and to a lesser extent the other proximal row of carpal bones on the radius.[6, 7] The opposite occurs with ulnar deviation. Distally the midcarpal row extends slightly during radial deviation, and flexes during ulnar deviation.[3] Thus restoring joint play into flexion and extension, as well as individual intercarpal mobility, is important in restoring radial deviation and ulnar deviation.

Most of the motion for radial deviation occurs at the midcarpal joint, whereas motion into ulnar deviation appears to be divided more equally between the two joints.[8, 11] When radial and ulnar deviation are being restored, emphasis therefore should be placed on achieving the appropriate balance of motion between the two rows.

THUMB FLEXION AND EXTENSION

The trapeziometacarpal joint is primarily responsible for thumb motion and is of utmost importance in hand function. The trapezium is flexed, abducted, and rotated internally in relation to the other carpal bones;[2] thus the trapeziometacarpal joint does not lie in the same plane as that of the fingers. Flexion and extension therefore take place in a plane approximately parallel to the plane of the hand. The trapeziometacarpal joint is a sellar joint, with the trapezium convex in a radial to ulnar direction. The glide to restore both flexion and extension therefore occurs in the same direction as the restriction. Flexion and extension also take place at the metacarpophalangeal and interphalangeal joints of the thumb, both of which are convex proximally and concave distally.

THUMB ABDUCTION AND ADDUCTION

The trapeziometacarpal joint is primarily responsible for abduction and adduction, although a small amount of abduction and adduction takes place at the metacarpophalangeal joint. Abduction and adduction occur in a plane approximately perpendicular to the plane of the hand. The trapezium is concave on a convex metacarpal in a volar to dorsal direction; therefore gliding takes place opposite the restriction. The distal aspect of the metacarpal is convex on a concave phalanx.

OPPOSITION

Opposition takes place at both the trapeziometacarpal and metacarpophalangeal articulations,[2] although most of this motion occurs at the trapeziometacarpal joint. Opposition at the trapeziometacarpal joint is thought to be a combination of flexion and medial rotation, and retroposition a combination of extension and lateral rotation,[9] although some authors regard abduction also as a component of opposition, and adduction of retroposition.[2, 11] A fair amount of ligamentous laxity must be present for the rotational component of opposition to occur. Restoring accessory motion in all planes of motion facilitates restoration of opposition.

ARCHING OF HAND

The articulations between the trapezoid and the second metacarpal and between the capitate and third metacarpal are extremely immobile, whereas the hamate and fourth and fifth metacarpal bones have relatively more movement. Similarly, the second and third metacarpals are relatively immobile in relation to each other, whereas movement of the third metacarpal on the fourth and of the fourth metacarpal on the fifth is greater. Restoring the appropriate motion between all these articulations facilitates arching of the hand, which is an important component of grasp.

FINGER FLEXION AND EXTENSION

Metacarpophalangeal movement at digits 2 through 5 occurs such that finger flexion accompanies adduction during grasp and extension accompanies abduction with opening of the hand. Interphalangeal motion, which also is necessary for grasp and release, involves primarily flexion and extension. All of these joints are comprised of a convex proximal and a concave distal articulation; thus oscillations should occur in the direction of the restriction.

FINGER ABDUCTION AND ADDUCTION

Abduction and adduction of the fingers take place at the metacarpophalangeal joints of digits 2 through 5. These joint surfaces are convex proximally and concave distally.

Radiocarpal and Ulnocarpal Joints

Osteokinematic degrees of freedom:	3 motions:
	   Flexion/extension
	   Radial/ulnar deviation
	   Pronation/supination

Ligaments:	Ulnar collateral ligament Radial collateral ligament Palmar radiocarpal ligaments Dorsal radiocarpal ligaments Intercarpal ligaments
Joint orientation:	Radius and ulna: Caudal, ventral, ulnar Carpals: Cranial, dorsal, radial
Type of joint:	Synovial
Articular surface anatomy:	Ovoid Radius and ulna: Concave Carpals: Convex
Resting position:	Neutral with slight ulnar deviation
Close-packed position:	Full extension
Capsular pattern of restriction:	Limitation is equal in all directions

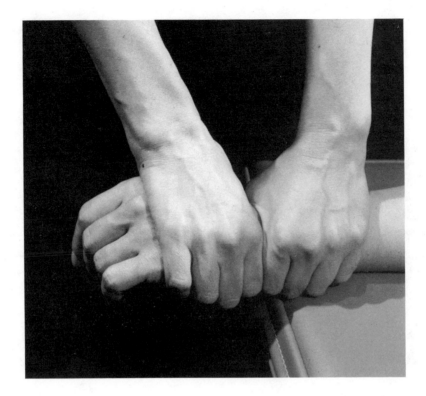

Distraction (Fig 4−2)

Purpose

- To increase joint play in the radiocarpal and ulnocarpal joints
- To increase overall range of motion in the radiocarpal and ulnocarpal joints
- To decrease pain in the wrist
- To increase nutrition to articular structures

Positioning

1. The patient is sitting with the ventral aspect of the forearm on the table and the hand off the table.
2. The radiocarpal and ulnocarpal joints are in the resting position if conservative techniques are indicated or approximating the restricted range if more aggressive techniques are indicated.
3. The clinician is facing the radiocarpal and ulnocarpal joints.
4. The stabilizing hand grips the distal radius and ulna from the dorsal side.
5. The manipulating hand grips the proximal row of carpals from the dorsal side.

Procedure

1. The stabilizing hand holds the radius and ulna to the table.
2. The manipulating hand moves the proximal row of carpals distally.

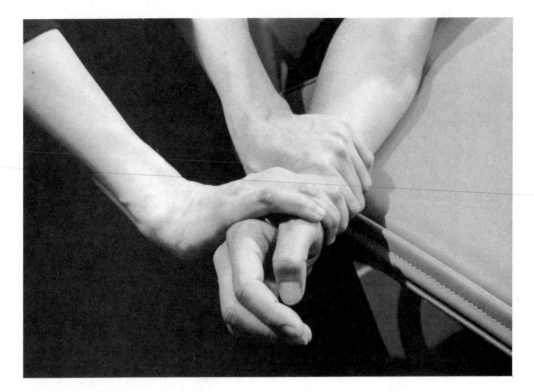

Dorsal Glide: (Fig 4–3)

Purpose

- To increase joint play in the radiocarpal and ulnocarpal joints
- To increase range of motion into wrist flexion
- To decrease pain in the wrist
- To increase nutrition to articular structures

Positioning

1. The patient is sitting with the ulnar aspect of the forearm on the table and the hand off the table.
2. The radiocarpal and ulnocarpal joints are in the resting position if conservative techniques are indicated or approximating the restricted range if more aggressive techniques are indicated.
3. The clinician is facing the radiocarpal and ulnocarpal joints.
4. The stabilizing hand grips the distal radius and ulna from the dorsal side.
5. The manipulating hand grips the proximal row of carpals from the dorsal side.

Procedure

1. The stabilizing hand holds the radius and ulna to the table.
2. The manipulating hand glides the proximal row of carpals in a dorsal direction.

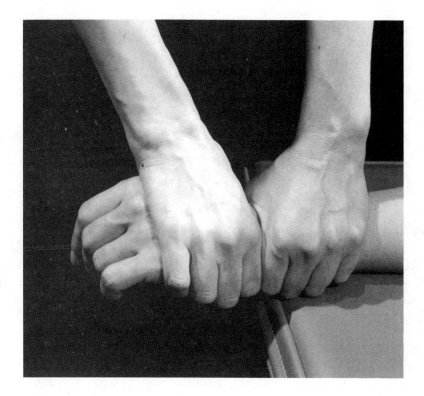

Ventral Glide (Fig 4–4)

Purpose

- To increase joint play in the radiocarpal and ulnocarpal joints
- To increase range of motion into wrist extension
- To decrease pain in the wrist
- To increase nutrition to articular structures

Positioning

1. The patient is sitting with the ventral aspect of the forearm on the table and the hand off the table.
2. The radiocarpal and ulnocarpal joints are in the resting position if conservative techniques are indicated or approximating the restricted range if more aggressive techniques are indicated.
3. The clinician is facing the radiocarpal and ulnocarpal joints.
4. The stabilizing hand grips the distal radius and ulna from the dorsal side.
5. The manipulating hand grips the proximal row of carpals from the dorsal side.

Procedure

1. The stabilizing hand holds the radius and ulna to the table.
2. The manipulating hand glides the proximal row of carpals in a volar direction.

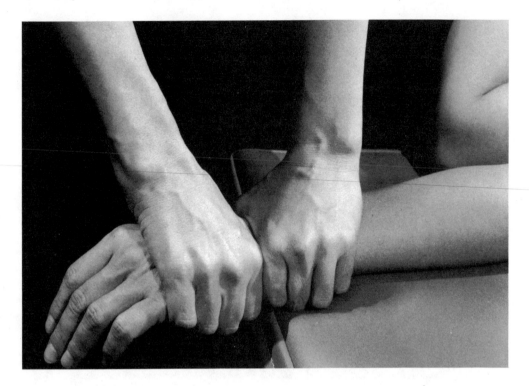

Radial Glide (Fig 4–5)

Purpose

- To increase joint play in the radiocarpal and ulnocarpal joints
- To increase range of motion into wrist ulnar deviation
- To decrease pain in the wrist
- To increase nutrition to articular structures

Positioning

1. The patient is sitting with the ventral aspect of the forearm on the table and the hand off the table.
2. The radiocarpal and ulnocarpal joints are in the resting position if conservative techniques are indicated or approximating the restricted range if more aggressive techniques are indicated.
3. The clinician is facing the radiocarpal and ulnocarpal joints.
4. The stabilizing hand grips the distal radius and ulna from the dorsal side.
5. The manipulating hand grips the proximal row of carpals from the ulnar side.

Procedure

1. The stabilizing hand holds the radius and ulna to the table.
2. The manipulating hand glides the proximal row of carpals in a radial direction.

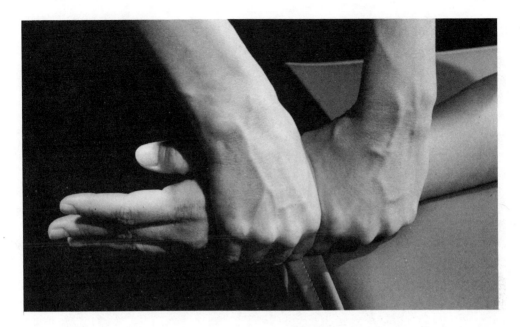

Ulnar Glide (Fig 4–6)

Purpose

- To increase joint play in the radiocarpal and ulnocarpal joints
- To increase range of motion into wrist radial deviation
- To decrease pain in the wrist
- To increase nutrition to articular structures

Positioning

1. The patient is sitting with the ulnar aspect of the forearm on the table and the hand off the table.
2. The radiocarpal and ulnocarpal joints are in the resting position if conservative techniques are indicated or approximating the restricted range if more aggressive techniques are indicated.
3. The clinician is facing the radial aspect of the radiocarpal joint.
4. The stabilizing hand grips the distal radius and ulna from the dorsal side.
5. The manipulating hand grips the proximal row of carpals from the radial side.

Procedure

1. The stabilizing hand holds the radius and ulna to the table.
2. The manipulating hand glides the proximal row of carpals in an ulnar direction.

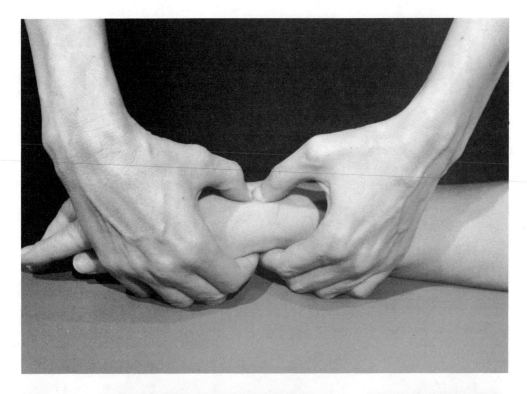

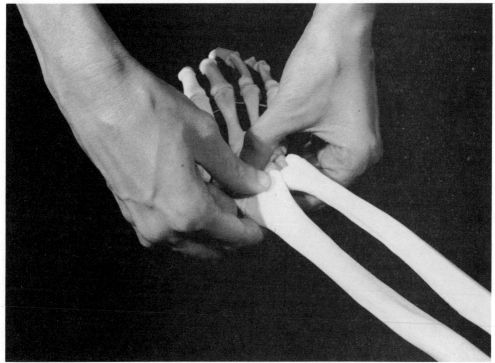

Specific Manipulations: For Restricted Extension (Figs 4–7, 4–8)

Purpose

- To increase joint play in the radiocarpal and ulnocarpal joints
- To increase range of motion into wrist extension
- To increase range of motion into supination, when the triquetrium is being manipulated in a volar direction on the ulna
- To decrease pain in the wrist
- To increase nutrition to articular structures

Positioning

1. The patient is sitting with the ventral aspect of the forearm on the table and the hand off the table.
2. The radiocarpal and ulnocarpal joints are in the resting position if conservative techniques are indicated or approximating the restricted range if more aggressive techniques are indicated.
3. The clinician is facing the radiocarpal and ulnocarpal joints.
4. The stabilizing hand grips the distal radius or ulna with the thumb on the dorsal surface and the index finger on the ventral surface.
5. Additional stabilization can be achieved by holding the patient's hand against the clinician's trunk.
6. The manipulating hand grips the proximal carpal bone with the thumb on the dorsal surface and the index finger on the volar surface.

Procedure

1. The stabilizing hand holds the radius or ulna in position.
2. The manipulating hand glides the scaphoid in a volar direction on the radius, the lunate in a volar direction on the radius, and the triquetrium in a volar direction on the disc.

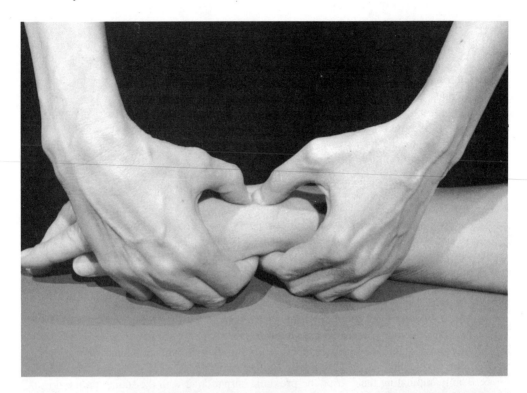

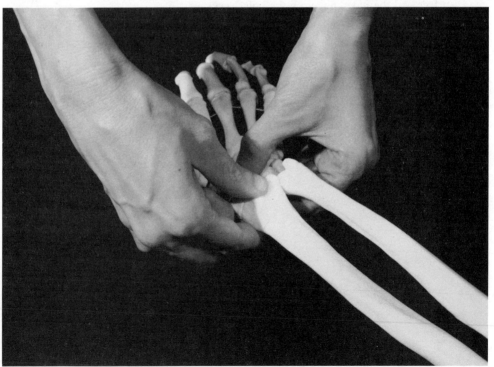

Specific Manipulations: For Restricted Flexion (Figs 4–9, 4–10)

Purpose

- To increase joint play in the radiocarpal and ulnocarpal joints
- To increase range of motion into wrist flexion
- To reduce a volar positional fault of the lunate, when the lunate is being manipulated dorsally on the radius
- To increase range of motion into pronation, when the triquetrium is being manipulated dorsally on the ulna
- To decrease pain in the wrist
- To increase nutrition to articular structures

Positioning

1. The patient is sitting with the ventral aspect of the forearm on the table and the hand off the table.
2. The radiocarpal and ulnocarpal joints are in the resting position if conservative techniques are indicated or approximating the restricted range if more aggressive techniques are indicated.
3. The clinician is facing the radiocarpal and ulnocarpal joints.
4. The stabilizing hand grips the distal radius or ulna with the thumb on the dorsal surface and the index finger on the ventral surface.
5. Additional stabilization can be achieved by holding the patient's hand against the clinician's trunk.
6. The manipulating hand grips the proximal carpal bone with the thumb on the dorsal surface and the index finger on the volar surface.

Procedure

1. The stabilizing hand holds the radius or ulna in position.
2. The manipulating hand glides the scaphoid in a dorsal direction on the radius, the lunate in a dorsal direction on the radius, and the triquetrium in a dorsal direction on the disc.

Specific Manipulations: Proximal Row Intercarpal Manipulations

Purpose

- To increase joint play between the proximal row of carpal bones
- To decrease pain in the wrist
- To increase nutrition to articular structures

Positioning

1. The patient is sitting with the ventral aspect of the forearm on the table and the hand off the table.
2. The radiocarpal and ulnocarpal joints are in the resting position if conservative techniques are indicated or approximating the restricted range if more aggressive techniques are indicated.
3. The clinician is facing the radiocarpal and ulnocarpal joints.

4. The stabilizing hand grips the one carpal bone with the thumb on the dorsal surface and the index finger on the volar surface.
5. Additional stabilization can be achieved by holding the patient's hand against the clinician's trunk.
6. The manipulating hand grips the other carpal bone with the thumb on the dorsal surface and the index finger on the volar surface.

Procedure

1. The stabilizing hand holds the one carpal bone in position.
2. The manipulating hand glides the scaphoid in a dorsal direction on the lunate, the scaphoid in a volar direction on the lunate, the triquetrium in a dorsal direction on the lunate, the triquetrium in a volar direction on the lunate. The pisiform is glided in a lateral direction on the triquetrium, and in a medial direction on the triquetrium.

Midcarpal Joints: Scaphoid/Trapezium, Trapezoid and Scaphoid, Lunate and Triquetrium/Capitate and Hamate

Osteokinematic degrees of freedom:	2 motions:
	Flexion/extension
	Radial deviation/ulnar deviation
Ligaments:	Radial collateral ligament
	Dorsal radiocarpal ligament
	Volar radiocarpal ligament
	Intercarpal ligament
Joint orientation:	Proximal row: Caudal
	Distal row: Cranial
Type of joint:	Synovial
Articular surface anatomy:	Scaphoid/trapezium and trapezoid: Sellar
	Scaphoid:
	Convex ventral to dorsal (flexion/extension)
	Concave radial to ulnar (radial/ulnar deviation)
	Trapezium and trapezoid:
	Concave ventral to dorsal (flexion/extension)
	Convex radial to ulnar (radial/ulnar deviation)
	Scaphoid, lunate, triquetrium/capitate, hamate: Ovoid
	Scaphoid, lunate, triquetrium: Concave
	Capitate, hamate: Convex
Resting position:	Neutral or slight flexion with slight ulnar deviation
Close-packed position:	Full extension
Capsular pattern of restriction:	Limitation is equal in all directions

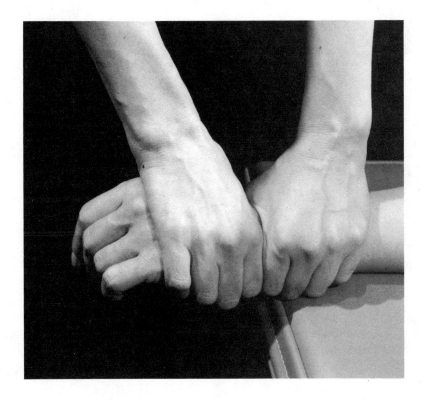

Distraction (Fig 4–11)

Purpose

- To increase joint play in the midcarpal joint
- To increase overall range of motion in the midcarpal joint
- To decrease pain in the wrist
- To increase nutrition to articular structures

Positioning

1. The patient is sitting with the ventral aspect of the forearm on the table and the hand off the table.
2. The midcarpal joint is in the resting position if conservative techniques are indicated or approximating the restricted range if more aggressive techniques are indicated.
3. The clinician is facing the midcarpal joint.
4. The stabilizing hand grips the proximal row of carpals from the dorsal side.
5. The manipulating hand grips the distal row of carpals from the dorsal side.

Procedure

1. The stabilizing hand holds the proximal row of carpals in position.
2. The manipulating hand moves the distal row of carpals distally.

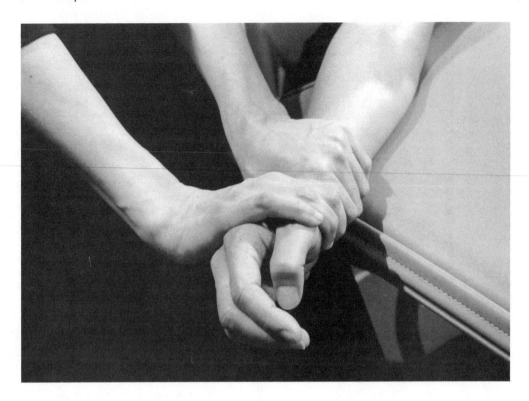

Dorsal Glide: (Fig 4–12)

Purpose

- To increase joint play in the midcarpal joint
- To increase range of motion into wrist flexion and extension
- To decrease pain in the wrist
- To increase nutrition to articular structures

Positioning

1. The patient is sitting with the ulnar aspect of the forearm on the table and the hand off the table.
2. The midcarpal joint is in the resting position if conservative techniques are indicated or approximating the restricted range if more aggressive techniques are indicated.
3. The clinician is facing the midcarpal joint.
4. The stabilizing hand grips the proximal row of carpals from the dorsal side.
5. The manipulating hand grips the distal row of carpals from the dorsal side.

Procedure

1. The stabilizing hand holds the proximal row of carpals in position.
2. The manipulating hand glides the distal row of carpals in a dorsal direction.

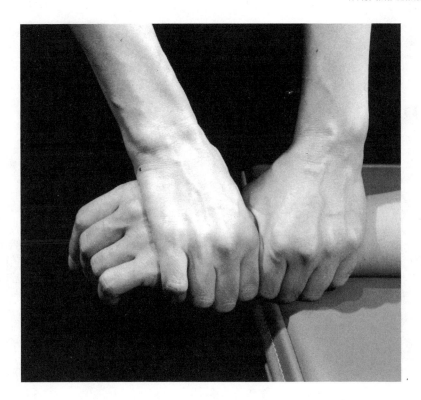

Ventral Glide (Fig 4–13)

Purpose

- To increase joint play in the midcarpal joint
- To increase range of motion into wrist flexion and extension
- To decrease pain in the wrist
- To increase nutrition to articular structures

Positioning

1. The patient is sitting with the ventral aspect of the forearm on the table and the hand off the table.
2. The midcarpal joint is in the resting position if conservative techniques are indicated or approximating the restricted range if more aggressive techniques are indicated.
3. The clinician is facing the midcarpal joint.
4. The stabilizing hand grips the proximal row of carpals from the dorsal side.
5. The manipulating hand grips the distal row of carpals from the dorsal side.

Procedure

1. The stabilizing hand holds the proximal row of carpals in position.
2. The manipulating hand glides the distal row of carpals in a ventral direction.

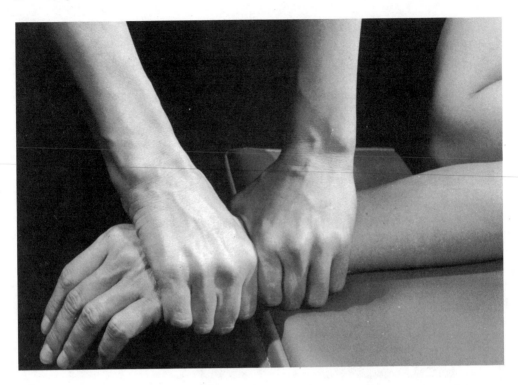

Radial Glide (Fig 4–14)

Purpose

- To increase joint play in the midcarpal joint
- To increase range of motion into wrist ulnar deviation
- To decrease pain in the wrist
- To increase nutrition to articular structures

Positioning

1. The patient is sitting with the ventral aspect of the forearm on the table and the hand off the table.
2. The midcarpal joint is in the resting position if conservative techniques are indicated or approximating the restricted range if more aggressive techniques are indicated.
3. The clinician is facing the midcarpal joint.
4. The stabilizing hand grips the proximal row of carpals from the dorsal side.
5. The manipulating hand grips the distal row of carpals from the ulnar side.

Procedure

1. The stabilizing hand holds the proximal row of carpals in position.
2. The manipulating hand glides the distal row of carpals in a radial direction.

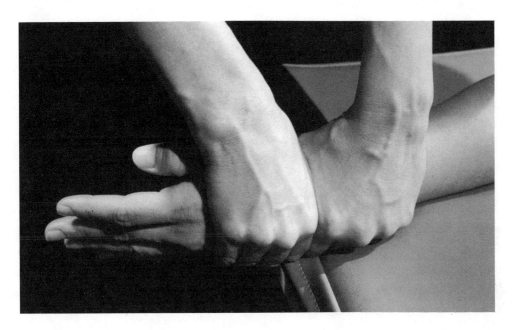

Ulnar Glide (Fig 4– 15)

Purpose

- To increase joint play in the midcarpal joint
- To increase range of motion into wrist radial deviation
- To decrease pain in the wrist
- To increase nutrition to articular structures

Positioning

1. The patient is sitting with the ulnar aspect of the forearm on the table and the hand off the table.
2. The midcarpal joint is in the resting position if conservative techniques are indicated or approximating the restricted range if more aggressive techniques are indicated.
3. The clinician is facing the midcarpal joint.
4. The stabilizing hand grips the proximal row of carpals from the dorsal side.
5. The manipulating hand grips the distal row of carpals from the radial side.

Procedure

1. The stabilizing hand holds the proximal row of carpals in position.
2. The manipulating hand glides the distal row of carpals in an ulnar direction.

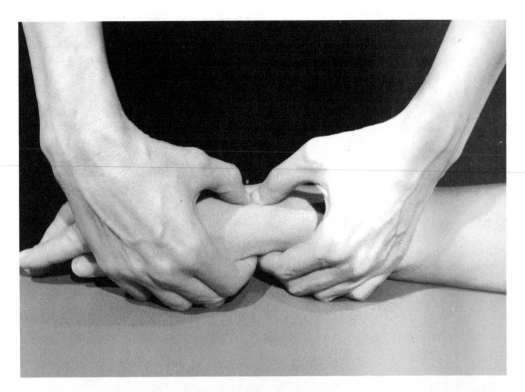

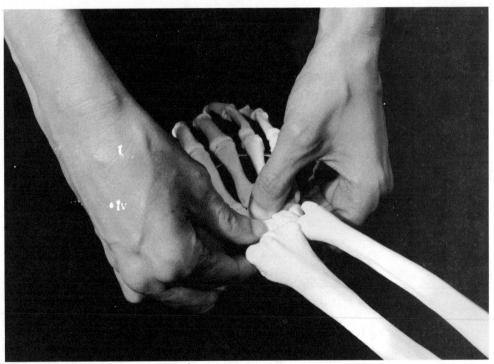

Specific Manipulations: For Restricted Extension (Figs 4–16, 4–17)

Purpose

- To increase joint play in the midcarpal joint
- To increase range of motion into wrist extension
- To decrease pain in the wrist
- To increase nutrition to articular structures

Positioning

1. The patient is sitting with the ventral aspect of the forearm on the table and the hand off the table.
2. The midcarpal joint is in the resting position if conservative techniques are indicated or approximating the restricted range if more aggressive techniques are indicated.
3. The clinician is facing the midcarpal joint.
4. The stabilizing hand grips the proximal carpal bone with the thumb on the dorsal surface and the index finger on the volar surface.
5. Additional stabilization can be achieved by holding the patient's hand against the clinician's trunk.
6. The manipulating hand grips the distal carpal bone with the thumb on the dorsal surface and the index finger on the volar surface.

Procedure

1. The stabilizing hand holds the proximal carpal bone in position.
2. The manipulating hand glides the trapezium and trapezoid in a dorsal direction on the scaphoid, the capitate in a volar direction on the scaphoid, the capitate in a volar direction on the lunate, and the hamate in a volar direction on the triquetrium.

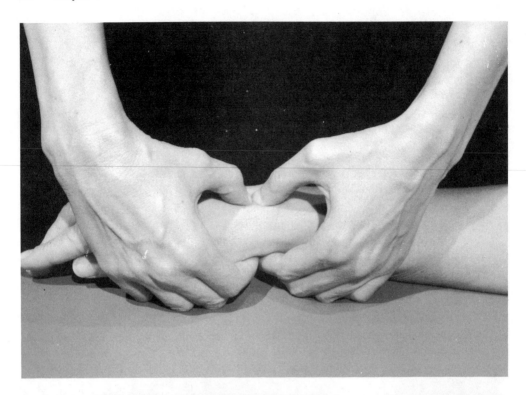

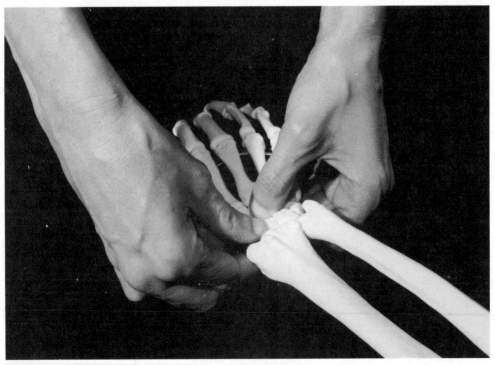

Specific Manipulations: For Restricted Flexion (Figs 4–18, 4–19)

Purpose

- To increase joint play in the midcarpal joint
- To increase range of motion into wrist flexion
- To decrease pain in the wrist
- To increase nutrition to articular structures

Positioning

1. The patient is sitting with the ventral aspect of the forearm on the table and the hand off the table.
2. The midcarpal joint is in the resting position if conservative techniques are indicated or approximating the restricted range if more aggressive techniques are indicated.
3. The clinician is facing the midcarpal joint.
4. The stabilizing hand grips the proximal carpal bone with the thumb on the dorsal surface and the index finger on the volar surface.
5. Additional stabilization can be achieved by holding the patient's hand against the clinician's trunk.
6. The manipulating hand grips the distal carpal bone with the thumb on the dorsal surface and the index finger on the volar surface.

Procedure

1. The stabilizing hand holds the proximal carpal bone in position.
2. The manipulating hand glides the trapezium and trapezoid in a volar direction on the scaphoid, the capitate in a dorsal direction on the scaphoid, the capitate in a dorsal direction on the lunate, and the hamate in a dorsal direction on the triquetrium.

Specific Manipulations: Distal Row Intercarpal Manipulations

Purpose

- To increase joint play between the distal row of carpals
- To decrease pain in the wrist
- To increase nutrition to articular structures

Positioning

1. The patient is sitting with the ventral aspect of the forearm on the table and the hand off the table.
2. The midcarpal joint is in the resting position if conservative techniques are indicated or approximating the restricted range if more aggressive techniques are indicated.
3. The clinician is facing the midcarpal joint.
4. The stabilizing hand grips the one carpal bone with the thumb on the dorsal surface and the index finger on the volar surface.
5. Additional stabilization can be achieved by holding the patient's hand against the clinician's trunk.
6. The manipulating hand grips the other carpal bone with the thumb on the dorsal surface and the index finger on the volar surface.

Procedure

1. The stabilizing hand holds the one carpal bone in position.
2. The manipulating hand glides the trapezoid in a dorsal direction on the capitate, the trapezoid in a volar direction on the capitate, the hamate in a dorsal direction on the capitate, and the hamate in a volar direction on the capitate.

Trapeziometacarpal Joint

Osteokinematic degrees of freedom:	3 motions:
	Flexion/extension
	Abduction/adduction
	Rotation
Ligaments:	Capsular ligament
Joint orientation:	Trapezium: Caudal, ventral, lateral
	First metacarpal: Cranial, dorsal, medial
Type of joint:	Synovial
Articular surface anatomy:	Sellar
	Trapezium:
	Convex radial to ulnar (flexion/extension)
	Concave dorsal to ventral (abduction/adduction)
	First metacarpal:
	Concave radial to ulnar (flexion/extension)
	Convex dorsal to ventral (abduction/adduction)
Resting position:	Midway between flexion and extension, and between abduction and adduction
Close-packed position:	Full opposition
Capsular pattern of restriction:	Abduction > extension

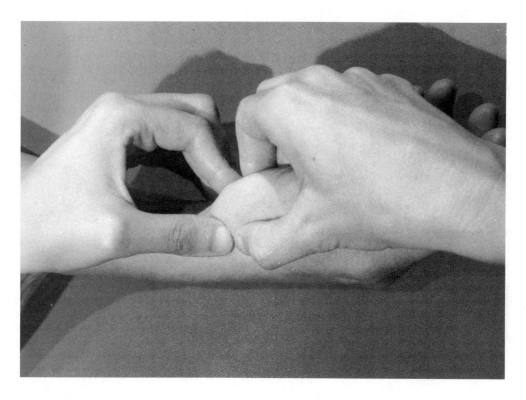

Distraction (Fig 4–20)

Purpose

- To increase joint play in the trapeziometacarpal joint
- To increase overall range of motion in the trapeziometacarpal joint
- To decrease pain in the trapeziometacarpal joint
- To increase nutrition to articular structures

Positioning

1. The patient is sitting with the ulnar aspect of the forearm on the table.
2. The trapeziometacarpal joint is in the resting position if conservative techniques are indicated or approximating the restricted range if more aggressive techniques are indicated.
3. The clinician is facing the trapeziometacarpal joint.
4. The stabilizing hand grips the trapezium with the thumb on the dorsal surface and the index finger on the volar surface.
5. Additional stabilization can be achieved by holding the patient's hand against the clinician's trunk.
6. The manipulating hand grips the proximal metacarpal with the thumb on the dorsal surface and the index finger on the volar surface.

Procedure

1. The stabilizing hand holds the trapezium in position.
2. The manipulating hand moves the metacarpal distally.

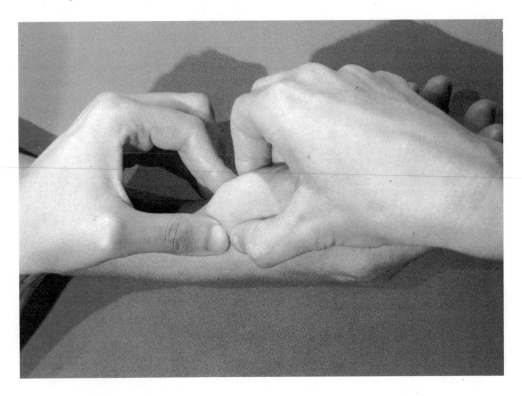

Dorsal Glide (Fig 4–21)

Purpose

- To increase joint play in the trapeziometacarpal joint
- To increase range of motion into trapeziometacarpal abduction
- To decrease pain in the trapeziometacarpal joint
- To increase nutrition to articular structures

Positioning

1. The patient is sitting with the ulnar aspect of the forearm on the table.
2. The trapeziometacarpal joint is in the resting position if conservative techniques are indicated or approximating the restricted range if more aggressive techniques are indicated.
3. The clinician is facing the trapeziometacarpal joint.
4. The stabilizing hand grips the trapezium with the thumb on the dorsal surface and the index finger on the volar surface.
5. Additional stabilization can be achieved by holding the patient's hand against the clinician's trunk.
6. The manipulating hand grips the proximal metacarpal with the thumb on the dorsal surface and the index finger on the volar surface.

Procedure

1. The stabilizing hand holds the trapezium in position.
2. The manipulating hand glides the metacarpal in a dorsal direction.

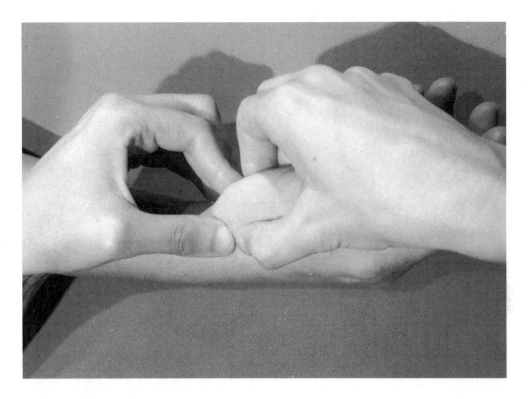

Volar Glide (Fig 4–22)

Purpose

- To increase joint play in the trapeziometacarpal joint
- To increase range of motion into trapeziometacarpal adduction
- To decrease pain in the trapeziometacarpal joint
- To increase nutrition to articular structures

Positioning

1. The patient is sitting with the ventral aspect of the forearm on the table.
2. The trapeziometacarpal joint is in the resting position if conservative techniques are indicated or approximating the restricted range if more aggressive techniques are indicated.
3. The clinician is facing the trapeziometacarpal joint.
4. The stabilizing hand grips the trapezium with the thumb on the dorsal surface and the index finger on the volar surface.
5. Additional stabilization can be achieved by holding the patient's hand against the clinician's trunk.
6. The manipulating hand grips the proximal metacarpal with the thumb on the dorsal surface and the index finger on the volar surface.

Procedure

1. The stabilizing hand holds the trapezium in position.
2. The manipulating hand glides the metacarpal in a volar direction.

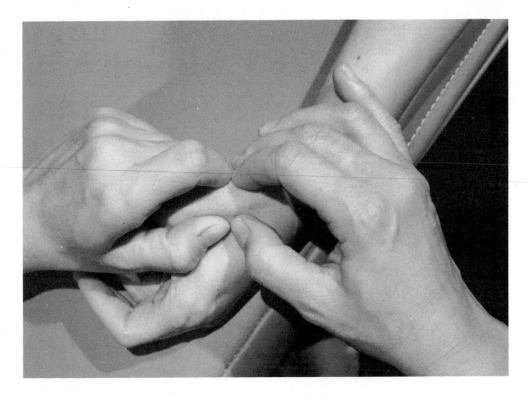

Radial Glide (Fig 4–23)

Purpose

- To increase joint play in the trapeziometacarpal joint
- To increase range of motion into trapeziometacarpal extension
- To decrease pain in the trapeziometacarpal joint .
- To increase nutrition to articular structures

Positioning

1. The patient is sitting with the ventral aspect of the forearm on the table.
2. The trapeziometacarpal joint is in the resting position if conservative techniques are indicated or approximating the restricted range if more aggressive techniques are indicated.
3. The clinician is facing the trapeziometacarpal joint.
4. The stabilizing hand grips the trapezium with the thumb on the dorsal surface and the index finger on the volar surface.
5. Additional stabilization can be achieved by holding the patient's hand against the clinician's trunk.
6. The manipulating hand grips the proximal metacarpal on the radial and ulnar surfaces.

Procedure

1. The stabilizing hand holds the trapezium in position.
2. The manipulating hand glides the metacarpal in a radial direction.

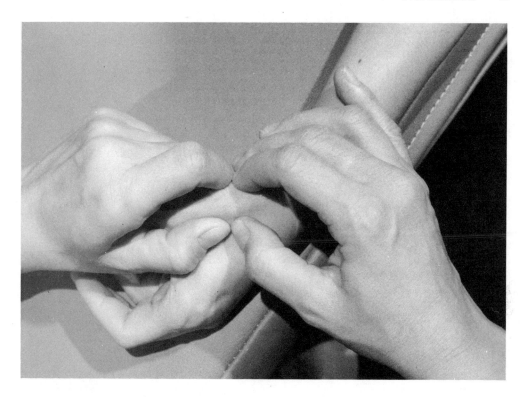

Ulnar Glide (Fig 4–24)

Purpose

- To increase joint play in the trapeziometacarpal joint
- To increase range of motion into trapeziometacarpal flexion
- To decrease pain in the trapeziometacarpal joint
- To increase nutrition to articular structures

Positioning

1. The patient is sitting with the ulnar aspect of the forearm on the table.
2. The trapeziometacarpal joint is in the resting position if conservative techniques are indicated or approximating the restricted range if more aggressive techniques are indicated.
3. The clinician is facing the trapeziometacarpal joint.
4. The stabilizing hand grips the trapezium with the thumb on the dorsal surface and the index finger on the volar surface.
5. Additional stabilization can be achieved by holding the patient's hand against the clinician's trunk.
6. The manipulating hand grips the proximal metacarpal on the radial and ulnar surfaces.

Procedure

1. The stabilizing hand holds the trapezium in position.
2. The manipulating hand glides the metacarpal in an ulnar direction.

Carpometacarpal Joints 2 Through 5

Osteokinematic degrees of freedom:	1 motion: Flexion/extension
Ligaments:	Dorsal ligament Palmar ligament Interosseous ligament
Joint orientation:	Carpals: Caudal Metacarpals: Cranial
Type of joint:	Synovial
Articular surface anatomy:	Ovoid Carpals: Convex Metacarpals: Concave
Resting position:	Midway between flexion and extension and slight ulnar deviation
Close-packed position:	Not described
Capsular pattern of restriction:	Equal in all directions

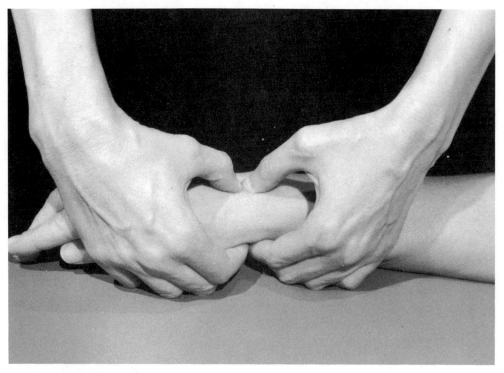

Distraction (Fig 4–25)

Purpose

- To increase joint play in the carpometacarpal joints of digits 2 through 5
- To increase overall range of motion in the carpometacarpal joints of digits 2 through 5
- To decrease pain in the carpometacarpal joints of digits 2 through 5
- To increase nutrition to articular structures

Positioning

1. The patient is sitting or supine with the palm down.
2. The joint is in the resting position.
3. The clinician is facing the carpometacarpal joints.
4. The stabilizing hand grips the carpal bone of the joint being manipulated with the thumb on the dorsal surface and the index finger on the volar surface.
5. Additional stabilization can be achieved by holding the patient's hand against the clinician's trunk.
6. The manipulating hand grips the base of the metacarpal of the joint being manipulated with the thumb on the dorsal surface and the index finger on the volar surface.

Procedure

1. The stabilizing hand holds the carpal bone in position.
2. The manipulating hand moves the second metacarpal distal on the trapezoid, the third metacarpal distal on the capitate, the fourth metacarpal distal on the hamate, and the fifth metacarpal distal on the hamate.
3. Movement in these joints is minimal, especially in the second and third carpometacarpal joints.

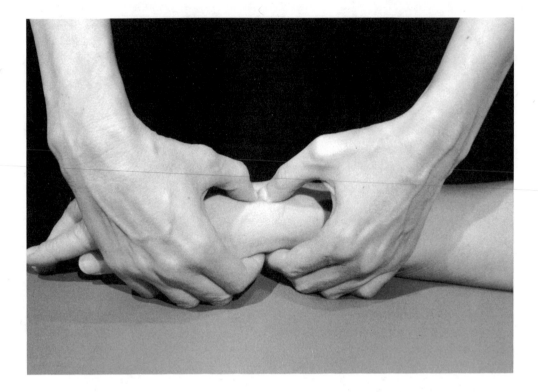

Dorsal Glide (Fig 4–26)

Purpose

- To increase joint play in the carpometacarpal joints of digits 2 through 5
- To increase range of motion into wrist extension of digits 2 through 5
- To decrease pain in the carpometacarpal joints of digits 2 through 5
- To increase nutrition to articular structures

Positioning

1. The patient is sitting or supine with the palm down.
2. The joint is in the resting position.
3. The clinician is facing the carpometacarpals.
4. The stabilizing hand grips the carpal bone of the joint being manipulated with the thumb on the dorsal surface and the index finger on the volar surface.
5. Additional stabilization can be achieved by holding the patient's hand against the clinician's trunk.
6. The manipulating hand grips the base of the metacarpal of the joint being manipulated with the thumb on the dorsal surface and the index finger on the volar surface.

Procedure

1. The stabilizing hand holds the carpal bone in position.
2. The manipulating hand glides the metacarpal in a dorsal direction.
3. Movement in these joints is minimal, especially in the second and third carpometacarpal joints.

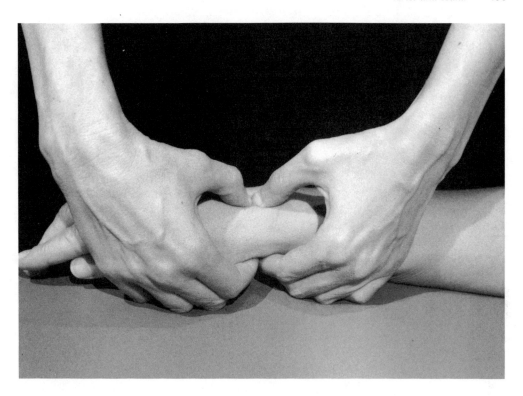

Volar Glide (Fig 4–27)

Purpose

- To increase joint play in the carpometacarpal joints of digits 2 through 5
- To increase range of motion into wrist flexion of digits 2 through 5
- To decrease pain in the carpometacarpal joints of digits 2 through 5
- To increase nutrition to articular structures

Positioning

1. The patient is sitting or supine with the palm down.
2. The joint is in the resting position.
3. The clinician is facing the carpometacarpal joints.
4. The stabilizing hand grips the carpal bone of the joint being manipulated with the thumb on the dorsal surface and the index finger on the volar surface.
5. Additional stabilization can be achieved by holding the patient's hand against the clinician's trunk.
6. The manipulating hand grips the base of the metacarpal being manipulated with the thumb on the dorsal surface and the index finger on the volar surface.

Procedure

1. The stabilizing hand holds the carpal bone in position.
2. The manipulating hand glides the metacarpal in a volar direction.
3. Movement in these joints is minimal, especially in the second and third carpometacarpal joints.

Intermetacarpal Joints Two Through Five

Osteokinematic degrees of freedom:	1 motion: Ventral/dorsal glide
Ligaments:	Palmar interosseous ligament Dorsal interosseous ligament
Joint orientation:	Medial metacarpal: Lateral Lateral metacarpal: Medial
Type of joint:	Synarthrosis
Articular surface anatomy:	Ovoid, plane Metacarpal III, Metacarpal IV ulnar border: Convex Metacarpal II ulnar border, Metacarpal IV and V radial border: Concave
Resting position:	Not described
Close-packed position:	None, not a synovial joint
Capsular pattern of restriction:	None, not a synovial joint

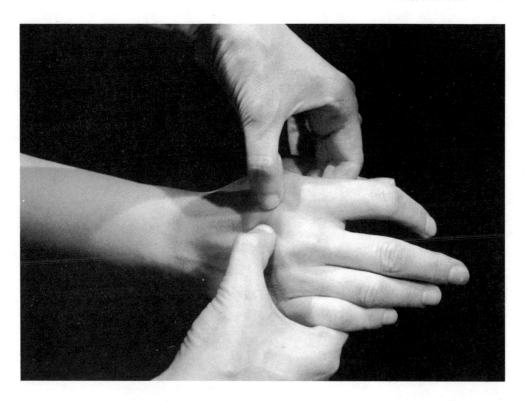

Dorsal Glide (Fig 4–28)

Purpose

- To increase joint play in the metacarpal articulations
- To increase range of motion into decreasing the arch of the hand
- To decrease pain in the palm of the hand

Positioning

1. The patient is sitting or supine with the palm down.
2. The joint is in the resting position.
3. The clinician is facing the metacarpal joints.
4. The stabilizing hand grips the midshaft of the one metacarpal with the thumb on the dorsal surface and the index finger on the volar surface.
5. Additional stabilization can be achieved by holding the patient's hand against the clinician's trunk.
6. The manipulating hand grips the midshaft of the other metacarpal with the thumb on the dorsal surface and the index finger on the volar surface.

Procedure

1. The stabilizing hand holds the metacarpal in position.
2. The manipulating hand glides the second metacarpal in a dorsal direction on the third metacarpal, the fourth metacarpal in a dorsal direction on the third metacarpal, and the fifth metacarpal in a dorsal direction on the fourth metacarpal.

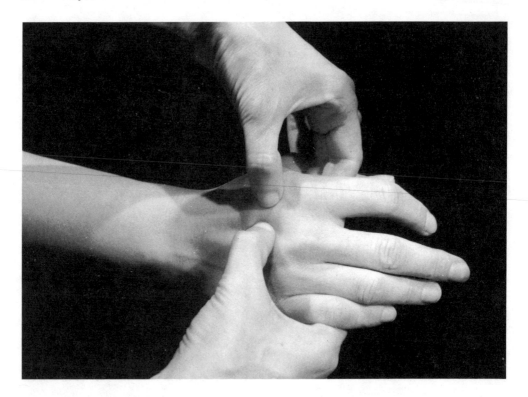

Volar Glide (Fig 4–29)

Purpose

- To increase joint play in the metacarpal articulations
- To increase range of motion into increasing the arch of the hand
- To decrease pain in the palm of the hand

Positioning

1. The patient is sitting or supine with the palm down.
2. The joint is in the resting position.
3. The clinician is facing the metacarpal joints.
4. The stabilizing hand grips the midshaft of the one metacarpal with the thumb on the dorsal surface and the index finger on the volar surface.
5. Additional stabilization can be achieved by holding the patient's hand against the clinician's trunk.
6. The manipulating hand grips the midshaft of the other metacarpal with the thumb on the dorsal surface and the index finger on the volar surface.

Procedure

1. The stabilizing hand holds the metacarpal in position.
2. The manipulating hand glides the second metacarpal in a volar direction on the third metacarpal, the fourth metacarpal in a volar direction on the third metacarpal, and the fifth metacarpal in a volar direction on the fourth metacarpal.

Metacarpophalangeal Joints 1 Through 5

Osteokinematic degrees of freedom:	3 motions
	Flexion/extension
	Radial/ulnar deviation
	Rotation
Ligaments:	Collateral ligament
	Palmar ligament
	Deep transverse ligament
Joint orientation:	Metacarpals: Caudal
	Phalanges: Cranial
Type of joint:	Synovial
Articular surface anatomy:	Ovoid
	Metacarpals: Convex
	Phalanges: Concave
Resting position:	First metacarpophalangeal joint: Slight flexion
	Metacarpophalangeal joints 2–5: Slight flexion with slight ulnar deviation
Close-packed position:	First metacarpophalangeal joint: Full extension
	Metacarpophalangeal joints 2–5: Full flexion
Capsular pattern of restriction:	Flexion > extension

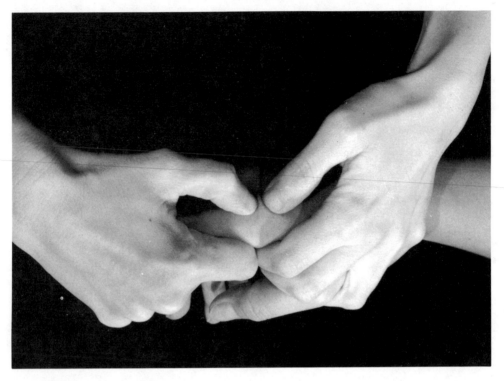

Distraction (Fig 4–30)

Purpose

- To increase joint play in the metacarpophalangeal joints
- To increase overall range of motion in the metacarpophalangeal joints
- To decrease pain in the metacarpophalangeal joints
- To increase nutrition to articular structures

Positioning

1. The patient is sitting or supine with the palm down.
2. The metacarpophalangeal joints are in the resting position if conservative techniques are indicated or approximating the restricted range if more aggressive techniques are indicated.
3. The clinician is facing the metacarpophalangeal joints.
4. The stabilizing hand grips the head of the metacarpal of the joint being manipulated with the thumb on the dorsal surface and the index finger on the volar surface.
5. Additional stabilization can be achieved by holding the patient's hand against the clinician's trunk.
6. The manipulating hand grips the proximal end of the proximal phalanx being manipulated with the thumb on the dorsal surface and the index finger on the volar surface.

Procedure

1. The stabilizing hand holds the metacarpal in position.
2. The manipulating hand moves the proximal phalanx distally.

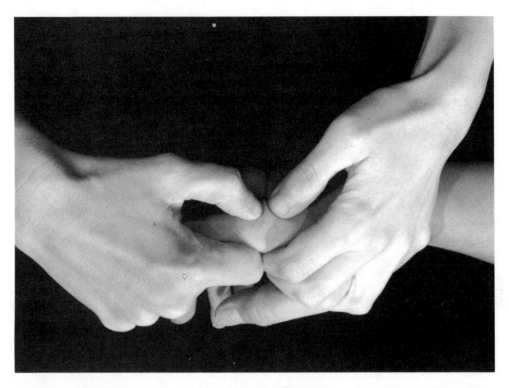

Dorsal Glide (First Metacarpophalangeal Joint Moves in a Radial Direction)
(Fig 4–31)

Purpose

- To increase joint play in the metacarpophalangeal joints
- To increase range of motion into metacarpophalangeal joint extension
- To decrease pain in the metacarpophalangeal joints
- To increase nutrition to articular structures

Positioning

1. The patient is sitting or supine with the palm down.
2. The metacarpophalangeal joints are in the resting position if conservative techniques are indicated or approximating the restricted range if more aggressive techniques are indicated.
3. The clinician is facing the metacarpophalangeal joints.
4. The stabilizing hand grips the head of the metacarpal of the joint being manipulated with the thumb on the dorsal surface and the index finger on the volar surface.
5. Additional stabilization can be achieved by holding the patient's hand against the clinician's trunk.
6. The manipulating hand grips the proximal end of the proximal phalanx being manipulated with the thumb on the dorsal surface and the index finger on the volar surface.

Procedure

1. The stabilizing hand holds the metacarpal in position.
2. The manipulating hand glides the proximal phalanx in a dorsal direction.

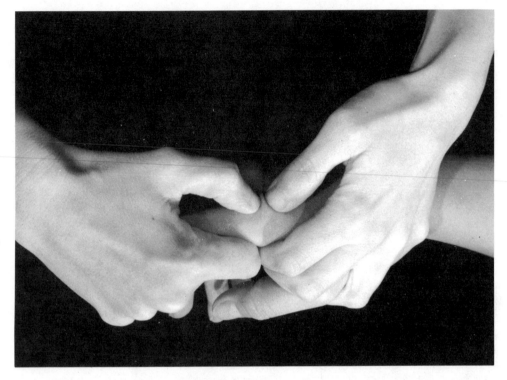

Volar Glide (First Metacarpophalangeal Joint Moves in an Ulnar Direction)
(Fig 4–32)

Purpose

- To increase joint play in the metacarpophalangeal joints
- To increase range of motion into metacarpophalangeal flexion
- To decrease pain in the metacarpophalangeal joints
- To increase nutrition to articular structures

Positioning

1. The patient is sitting or supine with the palm down.
2. The metacarpophalangeal joints are in the resting position if conservative techniques are indicated or approximating the restricted range if more aggressive techniques are indicated.
3. The clinician is facing the metacarpophalangeal joints.
4. The stabilizing hand grips the head of the metacarpal of the joint being manipulated with the thumb on the dorsal surface and the index finger on the volar surface.
5. Additional stabilization can be achieved by holding the patient's hand against the clinician's trunk.
6. The manipulating hand grips the proximal end of the proximal phalanx being manipulated with the thumb on the dorsal surface and the index finger on the volar surface.

Procedure

1. The stabilizing hand holds the metacarpal in position.
2. The manipulating hand glides the proximal phalanx in a volar direction.

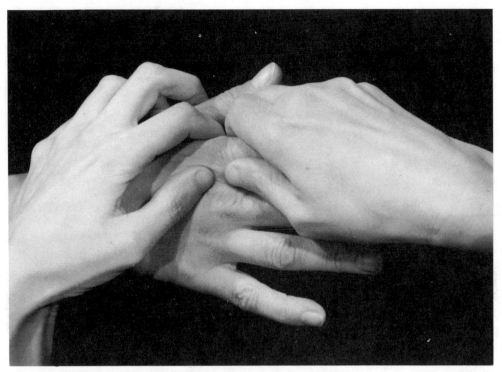

Radial Glide (First Metacarpophalangeal Joint Moves in a Volar Direction)
(Fig 4–33)

Purpose

- To increase joint play in the metacarpophalangeal joints
- To increase range of motion into the metacarpophalangeal joint, abduction of digits 1 and 2, radial abduction of digit 3, and adduction of digits 4 and 5.
- To decrease pain in the metacarpophalangeal joints
- To increase nutrition to articular structures

Positioning

1. The patient is sitting or supine with the palm down.
2. The metacarpophalangeal joints are in the resting position if conservative techniques are indicated or approximating the restricted range if more aggressive techniques are indicated.
3. The clinician is facing the metacarpophalangeal joint to be manipulated.
4. The stabilizing hand grips the head of the metacarpal of the joint being manipulated with the thumb on the dorsal surface and the index finger on the volar surface.
5. Additional stabilization can be achieved by holding the patient's hand against the clinician's trunk.
6. The manipulating hand grips the proximal end of the proximal phalanx being manipulated on the radial and ulnar surfaces.

Procedure

1. The stabilizing hand holds the metacarpal in position.
2. The manipulating hand glides the proximal phalanx radially.

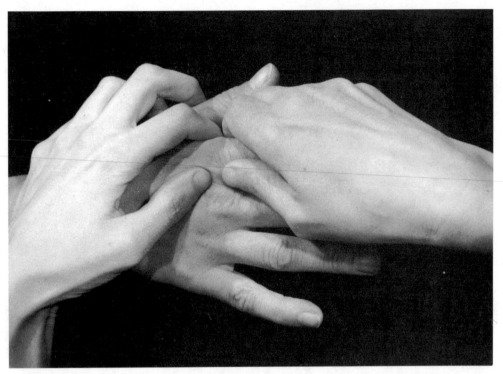

Ulnar Glide (First Metacarpophalangeal Joint Moves in a Dorsal Direction)
(Fig 4–34)

Purpose

- To increase joint play in the metacarpophalangeal joints
- To increase range of motion into the metacarpophalangeal joint, adduction of digits 1 and 2, ulnar abduction of digit 3, and abduction of digits 4 and 5.
- To decrease pain in the metacarpophalangeal joints
- To increase nutrition to articular structures

Positioning

1. The patient is sitting or supine with the palm down.
2. The metacarpophalangeal joints are in the resting position if conservative techniques are indicated or approximating the restricted range if more aggressive techniques are indicated.
3. The clinician is facing the metacarpophalangeal joint to be manipulated.
4. The stabilizing hand grips the head of the metacarpal of the joint being manipulated with the thumb on the dorsal surface and the index finger on the volar surface.
5. Additional stabilization can be achieved by holding the patient's hand against the clinician's trunk.
6. The manipulating hand grips the proximal end of the proximal phalanx being manipulated on the radial and ulnar surfaces.

Procedure

1. The stabilizing hand holds the metacarpal in position.
2. The manipulating hand glides the proximal phalanx in an ulnar direction.

Interphalangeal Joints One Through Five

Osteokinematic degrees of freedom:

1 motion:
    Flexion/extension

Ligaments:

Palmar ligament
    Medial collateral ligament
    Lateral collateral ligament
    Volar plate

Joint orientation:

Proximal phalanx: Caudal
    Distal phalanx: Cranial

Type of joint:

Synovial

Articular surface anatomy:

Sellar, functionally ovoid
Proximal phalanx: Convex ventral to dorsal
    (flexion/extension)
Distal phalanx: Concave ventral to dorsal
    (flexion/extension)

Resting position:

Proximal interphalangeal joints: 10 degrees flexion
Distal interphalangeal joints: 30 degrees flexion

Close-packed position:

Full extension

Capsular pattern of restriction:

Flexion > extension

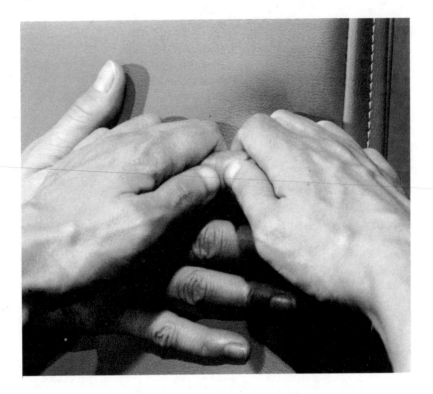

Distraction (Fig 4–35)

Purpose

- To increase joint play in the interphalangeal joints
- To increase overall range of motion in the interphalangeal joints
- To decrease pain in the interphalangeal joints
- To increase nutrition to articular structures

Positioning

1. The patient is sitting or supine with the palm down.
2. The interphalangeal joints are in the resting position if conservative techniques are indicated or approximating the restricted range if more aggressive techniques are indicated.
3. The clinician is facing the interphalangeal joints.
4. The stabilizing hand grips the distal end of the more proximal phalanx of the joint to be manipulated with the thumb on the dorsal surface and the index finger on the volar surface.
5. Additional stabilization can be achieved by holding the patient's hand against the clinician's trunk.
6. The manipulating hand grips the proximal end of the more distal phalanx of the joint to be manipulated with the thumb on the dorsal surface and the index finger on the volar surface.

Procedure

1. The stabilizing hand holds the proximal phalanx in position.
2. The manipulating hand moves the distal phalanx distally.
3. The use of a padded tongue depressor to manipulate may assist the clinician in directing a more precise manipulation.
4. Wearing surgical gloves may allow the clinician to obtain a stronger grip by reducing slippage against the patient's skin.

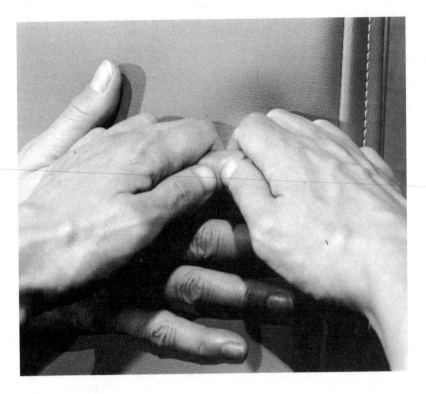

Dorsal Glide (Fig 4–36)

Purpose

- To increase joint play in the interphalangeal joints
- To increase range of motion into interphalangeal extension
- To decrease pain in the interphalangeal joints
- To increase nutrition to articular structures

Positioning

1. The patient is sitting or supine with the palm down.
2. The interphalangeal joints are in the resting position if conservative techniques are indicated or approximating the restricted range if more aggressive techniques are indicated.
3. The clinician is facing the interphalangeal joints.
4. The stabilizing hand grips the distal end of the more proximal phalanx of the joint to be manipulated with the thumb on the dorsal surface and the index finger on the volar surface.
5. Additional stabilization can be achieved by holding the patient's hand against the clinician's trunk.
6. The manipulating hand grips the proximal end of the more distal phalanx of the joint to be manipulated with the thumb on the dorsal surface and the index finger on the volar surface.

Procedure

1. The stabilizing hand holds the proximal phalanx in position.
2. The manipulating hand glides the distal phalanx in a dorsal direction.
3. The use of a padded tongue depressor to manipulate may assist the clinician in directing a more precise manipulation.
4. Wearing surgical gloves may allow the clinician to obtain a stronger grip by reducing slippage against the patient's skin.

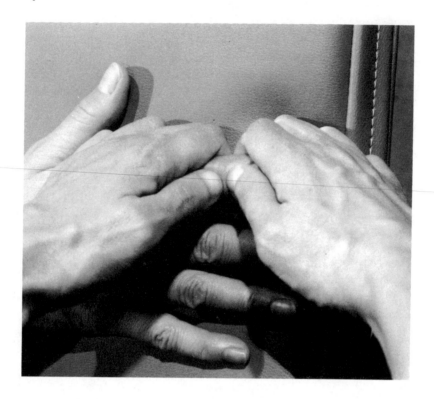

Volar Glide (Fig 4–37)

Purpose

- To increase joint play in the interphalangeal joints
- To increase range of motion into the interphalangeal flexion
- To decrease pain in the interphalangeal joints
- To increase nutrition to articular structures

Positioning

1. The patient is sitting or supine with the palm down.
2. The interphalangeal joints are in the resting position if conservative techniques are indicated or approximating the restricted range if more aggressive techniques are indicated.
3. The clinician is facing the interphalangeal joints.
4. The stabilizing hand grips the distal end of the more proximal phalanx of the joint to be manipulated with the thumb on the dorsal surface and the index finger on the volar surface.
5. Additional stabilization can be achieved by holding the patient's hand against the clinician's trunk.
6. The manipulating hand grips the proximal end of the more distal phalanx of the joint to be manipulated with the thumb on the dorsal surface and the index finger on the volar surface.

Procedure

1. The stabilizing hand holds the proximal phalanx in position.
2. The manipulating hand glides the distal phalanx in a volar direction.
3. The use of a padded tongue depressor to manipulate may assist the clinician in directing a more precise manipulation.
4. Wearing surgical gloves may allow the clinician to obtain a stronger grip by reducing slippage against the patient's skin.

REFERENCES

1. Brumfield RH, Champoux JA: A biomechanical study of normal functional wrist motion. *Clin Orthop* 1984; 187:23.
2. Cooney WP et al: The kinesiology of the thumb trapeziometacarpal joint. *J Bone Joint Surg* 1981; 63A:1371.
3. de Lange A, Kauer JMG, Huiskes R: Kinematic behavior of the human wrist joint: A roentgen-stereophotogrammetric analysis. *J Orthop Res* 1985; 3:56.
4. Hertling D, Kessler RM: The wrist and hand complex, in Hertling D, Kessler RM (eds): *Management of Common Musculoskeletal Disorders,* ed 2. Philadelphia, JB Lippincott, 1990.
5. Kauer JMG: Functional anatomy of the wrist. *Clin Orthop* 1980; 149:9.
6. Linscheid RL: Kinematic considerations of the wrist. *Clin Orthop* 1986; 202:27.
7. Ruby LK et al: Relative motion of selected carpal bones: A kinematic analysis of the normal wrist. *J Hand Surg* 1988; 13A:1.
8. Soderberg GL: *Kinesiology.* Baltimore, Williams & Wilkins, 1986.
9. Volz RG, Lieb M, Benjamin J: Biomechanics of the wrist. *Clin Orthop* 1980; 149:112.
10. Weber ER: Concepts governing the rotational shift of the intercalated segment of the carpus. *Orthop Clin North Am* 1984; 15:193.
11. Youm Y et al: Kinematics of the wrist. *J Bone Joint Surg* 1978; 60-A:423.

Figure **5—1**

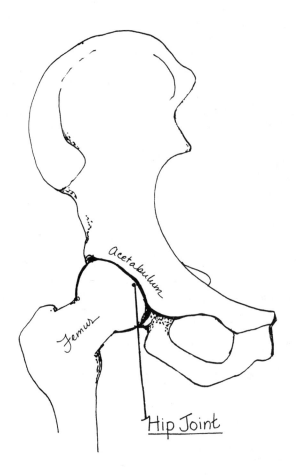

Hip Joint

Chapter 5 _____

Hip

The hip joint is a ball-and-socket joint with a compressed ventral-to-dorsal diameter. It deforms in weight bearing to increase congruency between the two joint surfaces.[2] Its construction is similar to that of the shoulder, but the hip is far more stable. This is due to negative intracapsular atmospheric pressure, a stronger joint capsule, a more spherical femoral head, and a deeper socket made even deeper by the labrum, which provides greater joint surface contact area. Arthrokinematic motion generally is thought to consist of gliding of the femoral sphere in the acetabular socket, although it has also been described as pivoting of the femoral head within the acetabulum.[3] This would require a greater amount of rolling motion, making range of motion techniques more effective than manipulation in restoring joint motion. Most functional activities occur between 0 and 120 degrees of flexion and between 0 and 20 degrees of both external rotation and abduction.[1]

FLEXION AND EXTENSION

Inasmuch as the acetabulum is concave on a convex femur, manipulations involving gliding of the femur are administered in a direction opposite that of motion being restored. Because of the oblique angulation of the acetabulum and the femoral angle of inclination, flexion is restored by dorsally gliding the femur, and extension by ventrally gliding the femur.

ABDUCTION AND ADDUCTION

Abduction is restored by caudally gliding the femur, and adduction by laterally gliding the femur.

ROTATION

External rotation is restored by ventrally gliding the femur, and internal rotation by dorsally and laterally gliding the femur. Internal rotation can be restored by performing the two glides separately or in combination with one another.

Hip Joint

Osteokinematic degrees of freedom:	3 motions: 　Flexion/extension 　Abduction/adduction 　Rotation
Ligaments:	Iliofemoral (Y) ligament Ischiofemoral ligament Pubofemoral ligament Ligamentum teres Zona orbicularis Transverse ligament
Joint orientation:	Acetabulum: Caudal, lateral, ventral Femur: Cranial, medial, ventral
Type of joint:	Synovial
Articular surface anatomy:	Ovoid Acetabulum: Concave Femur: Convex
Resting position:	30 degrees flexion, 30 degrees abduction, slight external rotation
Close-packed position:	Ligamentous: Full extension, abduction, and internal rotation Bony: 90 degrees flexion, slight abduction, and slight external rotation
Capsular pattern of restriction:	Flexion, abduction, internal rotation > extension, adduction, external rotation

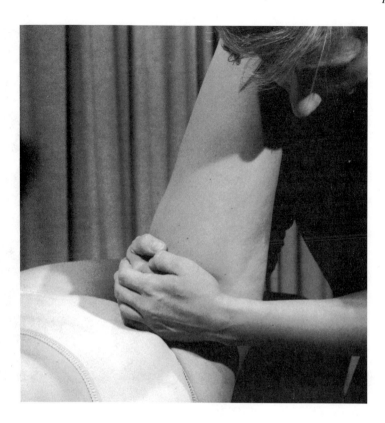

Distraction (Fig 5–2)

Purpose

- To increase joint play in the hip joint
- To increase overall range of motion in the hip joint
- To decrease pain in the hip joint
- To increase nutrition to articular structures

Positioning

1. The patient is supine with the leg positioned over the clinician's shoulder.
2. A belt may be wrapped around the patient's pelvis and the treatment table to help stabilize the pelvis.
3. The hip joint is positioned in as close to the resting position as possible if conservative techniques are indicated or approximating the restricted range if more aggressive techniques are indicated.
4. The clinician is at the patient's foot facing the patient's hip.
5. Both hands are positioned on the ventral and medial surfaces of the proximal thigh.

Procedure

1. Both hands move the femoral head away from the acetabulum at a 90-degree angle, thus imparting a caudal and lateral force to the hip joint.
2. The clinician's shoulder directs the femoral head in a ventral direction by elevating the scapula.

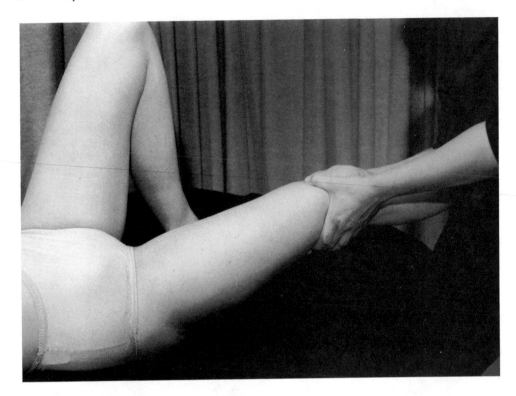

Caudal Glide (Fig 5–3)

Purpose

- To increase joint play in the hip joint
- To increase range of motion into hip abduction
- To decrease pain in the hip joint
- To increase nutrition to articular structures

Positioning

1. The patient is supine.
2. A belt may be wrapped around the patient's pelvis and the treatment table to help stabilize the pelvis.
3. The hip joint is positioned in the resting position if conservative techniques are indicated or approximating the restricted range if more aggressive techniques are indicated.
4. The clinician is standing at the patient's foot facing the patient's hip.
5. Both hands grip the distal thigh.

Procedure

1. Both hands glide the femoral head in a caudal direction as the clinician leans away from the joint.

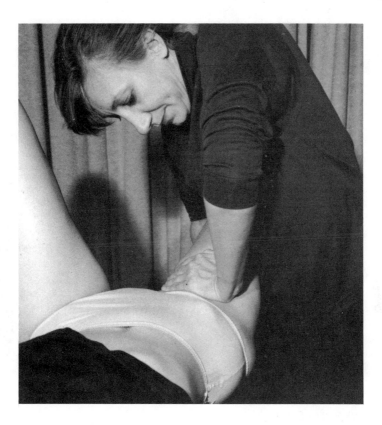

Dorsal Glide (Fig 5−4)

Purpose

- To increase joint play in the hip joint
- To increase range of motion into hip flexion
- To increase range of motion into hip internal rotation
- To decrease pain in the hip joint
- To increase nutrition to articular structures

Positioning

1. The patient is supine.
2. The hip joint is positioned in the resting position if conservative techniques are indicated or approximating the restricted range if more aggressive techniques are indicated.
3. The clinician is at the patient's knee facing the patient's hip.
4. The patient's leg is supported between the clinician's arm and trunk.
5. The manipulating hand is positioned on the ventral surface of the proximal thigh.
6. The guiding hand is positioned on the dorsal surface of the distal thigh.

Procedure

1. The manipulating hand glides the femur in a dorsal direction.
2. The guiding hand controls the position of the femur.

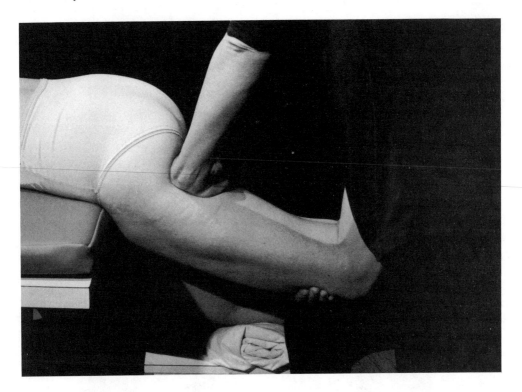

Ventral Glide (Fig 5–5)

Purpose

- To increase joint play in the hip joint
- To increase range of motion into hip extension
- To increase range of motion into hip external rotation
- To decrease pain in the hip joint
- To increase nutrition to articular structures

Positioning

1. The patient is prone with the leg off the treatment table.
2. A belt may be wrapped around the patient's thigh and the clinician's shoulder to help control the motion.
3. The hip joint is positioned in the resting position if conservative techniques are indicated or approximating the restricted range if more aggressive techniques are indicated.
4. The clinician is standing at the foot of the table facing the patient's hip.
5. The manipulating hand is positioned on the dorsal surface of the proximal thigh.
6. The guiding hand is positioned on the ventral surface of the distal thigh.

Procedure

1. The manipulating hand glides the femur in a ventral direction as the therapist leans on the patient's thigh.
2. The guiding hand controls the position of the thigh.

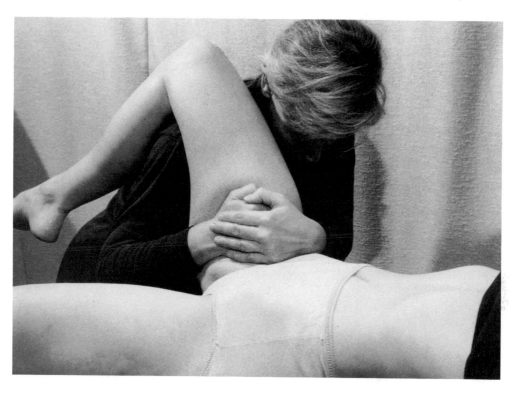

Lateral Glide (Fig 5—6)

Purpose

- To increase joint play in the hip joint
- To increase range of motion into hip internal rotation
- To increase range of motion into hip adduction
- To decrease pain in the hip joint
- To increase nutrition to articular structures

Positioning

1. The patient is supine with his leg positioned over the clinician's shoulder.
2. A belt may be wrapped around the patient's pelvis and treatment table to help stabilize the pelvis.
3. The hip joint is positioned in the resting position if conservative techniques are indicated or approximating the restricted range if more aggressive techniques are indicated.
4. The clinician is at the patient's side facing the patient's hip.
5. Both hands are positioned on the medial surface of the proximal thigh.

Procedure

1. Both hands glide the femur in a lateral direction.

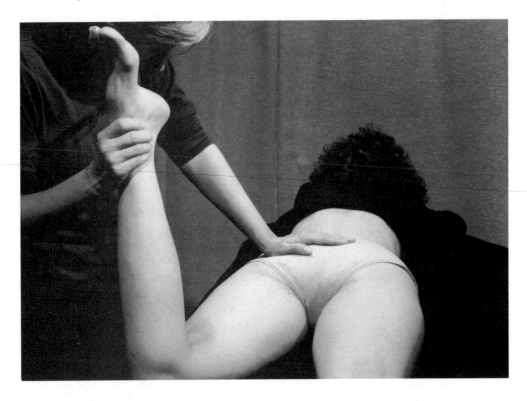

Dorsolateral Glide of the Femur on the Pelvis (Fig 5–7)

Purpose

- To increase joint play in the hip joint
- To increase range of motion into hip internal rotation
- To decrease pain in the hip joint
- To increase nutrition to articular structures

Positioning

1. The patient is prone with knees flexed to 90 degrees.
2. The hip joint is positioned in as close to resting position as possible if conservative techniques are indicated or approximating the restricted range if more aggressive techniques are indicated.
3. The clinician is at the patient's side facing the patient's hip.
4. The stabilizing hand grips the ankle and controls the amount of hip rotation.
5. The manipulating hand is positioned over the dorsal surface of the ilium.

Procedure

1. The stabilizing hand holds the leg in position.
2. The manipulating hand glides the pelvis in a ventromedial direction, thus imparting a dorsolateral force to the femur on the pelvis.
3. The sacroiliac joint must be examined prior to treatment, because the technique transmits some of the motion to this joint.

REFERENCES

1. Johnston RC, Smidt GL: Hip motion measurements for selected activities of daily living. *Clin Orthop* 1970; 72:205.
2. Radin EL: Biomechanics of the human hip. *Clin Orthop* 1980; 152:28.
3. Rydell N: Biomechanics of the hip-joint. *Clin Orthop* 1973; 92:6.

Figure 6 – 1

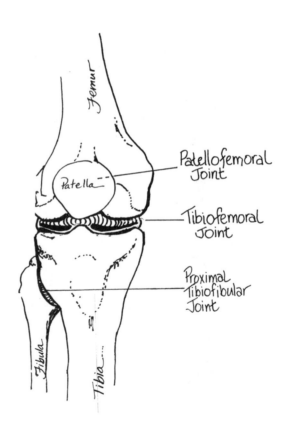

Knee Joints

Chapter 6

Knee

The knee joint consists of two sets of articulating surfaces, the tibiofemoral joint and the patellofemoral joint. To perform most activities of daily living, these two joints surfaces must permit at least 110 degrees of motion in the sagittal plane, 15 degrees in the frontal plane, and 15 degrees of rotation.[3, 4]

FLEXION AND EXTENSION

Flexion at the knee is accompanied by internal rotation and adduction of the tibia, and extension is accompanied by external rotation and abduction.[3] External rotation occurs during the last 30 degrees of extension. This rotational motion is produced by tightening of ligamentous structures and by muscular forces, as well as by the configuration of the two articular surfaces. Flexion is accompanied by dorsal gliding and rolling of the tibia on the femur, and extension by a similar ventral motion. The lateral femoral condyle moves more than two times farther than does the medial femoral condyle.[5] The relative ratio of rolling to gliding at the lateral joint is approximately equal, whereas medially, gliding is the predominant motion.[5] This partially explains why external rotation accompanies extension and internal rotation accompanies flexion. To restore normal knee biomechanics, it therefore may be necessary to ensure that a greater amount of motion exists laterally and that the appropriate amount of gliding relative to rolling is restored at both the medial and lateral articulations.

Oscillations are extremely important for restoring motion to the tibiofemoral joint. Most often the manipulations to increase knee motion involve dorsal and ventral gliding. Because the femur is a convex articulation on a concave tibia, the manipulation glide is in the direction of the restriction. Some clinicians perform medial and lateral gliding and gapping as well, because this is considered an accessory motion to all knee movements. Excessive medial and lateral motion is prevented by the spine of the tibia and its articulation into the femoral condylar notch.

The patellofemoral joint moves 5 to 7 cm cranially in the femoral groove as the knee extends. It is positioned laterally when the knee is in full flexion, glides medially as the knee begins to extend, and returns to a slightly more lateral position as the knee approaches full extension.[1, 2] The five facets on the dorsal side of the patella compose the patellar articulation with the femoral groove. The patellar surface is convex on a concave femur. The direction in which the patella is glided corresponds to the motion being restored, despite the fact that the moving bone is convex. This is because the ventral surface of the patella tilts in the direction opposite the restriction when the patella is glided in the direction of the restriction. A careful evaluation should precede lateral glide techniques, as this motion is sometimes hypermobile in dysfunctional knees, and if hypermobility is present, treatment with lateral gliding could cause the patella to sublux laterally. Conversely, dysfunction at the patellofemoral joint frequently results from decreased medial gliding.

Tibiofemoral Joint

Osteokinematic degrees of freedom:	2 motions:
	    Flexion/extension
	    Rotation

Ligaments:	Medial collateral ligament Lateral collateral ligament Anterior cruciate ligament Posterior cruciate ligament Oblique ligament Arcuate popliteal ligament
Joint orientation:	Femur: Caudal Tibia: Cranial
Type of joint:	Synovial
Articular surface anatomy:	Ovoid Femur: Convex Tibia: Concave
Resting position:	25 degrees of flexion
Close-packed position:	Full extension and external rotation
Capsular pattern of restriction:	Flexion > extension

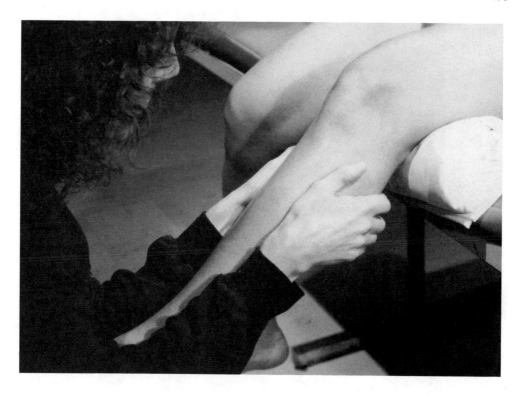

Distraction (Fig 6–2)

Purpose

- To increase joint play in the tibiofemoral joint
- To increase overall range of motion in the tibiofemoral joint
- To decrease pain in the knee
- To increase nutrition to articular structures

Positioning

1. The patient is sitting with the knee off the edge of the treatment table.
2. The tibiofemoral joint is positioned in the resting position if conservative techniques are indicated or approximating the restricted range if more aggressive techniques are indicated.
3. The clinician is at the patient's foot facing the patient's knee.
4. Both hands grip the distal tibia from the medial and lateral sides.
5. A specialized belt with a strap that wraps around the patient's tibia and a stirrup attachment for placement of the clinician's foot can be used to assist with distraction of the tibia.

Procedure

1. Both hands move the tibia distally.

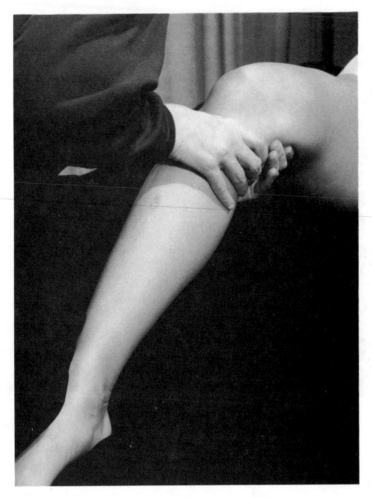

Dorsal Glide (Fig 6–3)

Purpose

- To increase joint play in the tibiofemoral joint
- To increase range of motion into knee flexion
- To decrease pain in the knee
- To increase nutrition to articular structures

Positioning

1. The patient is supine.
2. The tibiofemoral joint is positioned in the resting position if conservative techniques are indicated or approximating the restricted range if more aggressive techniques are indicated.
3. The clinician is at the patient's foot facing the patient's knee.
4. The stabilizing hand supports the femur from the dorsal side.
5. The manipulating hand grips the proximal tibia from the ventral side.

Procedure

1. The stabilizing hand holds the femur in position.
2. The manipulating hand glides the tibia in a dorsal direction.

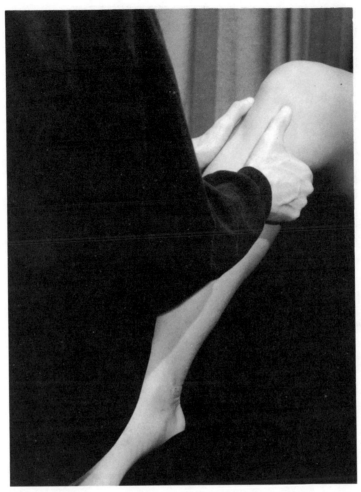

Ventral Glide of the Tibia on the Femur: First Technique (Fig 6–4)

Purpose

- To increase joint play in the tibiofemoral joint
- To increase range of motion into knee extension
- To decrease pain in the knee
- To increase nutrition to articular structures

Positioning

1. The patient is supine.
2. The tibiofemoral joint is positioned in the resting position if conservative techniques are indicated or approximating the restricted range if more aggressive techniques are indicated.
3. The clinician is at the patient's foot facing the patient's knee.
4. Both hands grip the proximal tibia from the dorsal side.

Procedure

1. Both hands glide the tibia in a ventral direction.

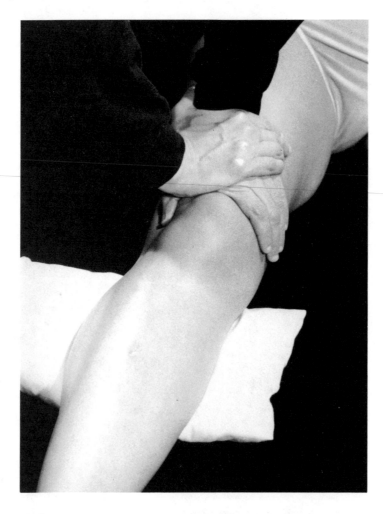

Ventral Glide of the Tibia on the Femur: Second Technique (Fig 6-5)

Purpose

- To increase joint play in the tibiofemoral joint
- To increase range of motion into knee extension
- To decrease pain in the knee
- To increase nutrition to articular structures

Positioning

1. The patient is supine.
2. The tibiofemoral joint is approximating the restricted range into extension.
3. The clinician is at the patient's side facing the tibiofemoral joint.
4. Both hands are positioned over the ventral surface of the distal femur.

Procedure

1. Both hands glide the femur in a dorsal direction, thus imparting a ventral force to the tibia on the femur.

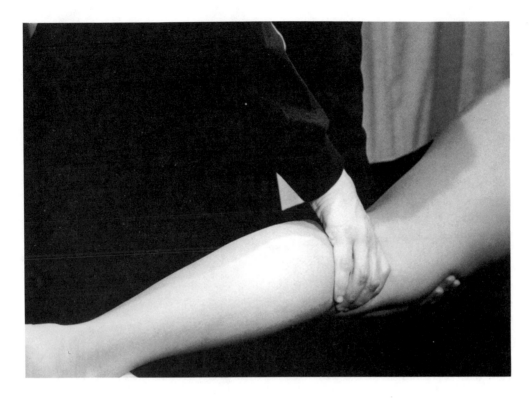

Ventral Glide of the Tibia on the Femur: Third Technique (Fig 6–6)

Purpose

- To increase joint play in the tibiofemoral joint
- To increase range of motion into knee extension
- To decrease pain in the knee
- To increase nutrition to articular structures

Positioning

1. The patient is prone.
2. The tibiofemoral joint is approximating the restricted range into extension.
3. The clinician is at the patient's side facing the tibiofemoral joint.
4. The stabilizing hand grips the distal femur from the ventral side.
5. The manipulating hand is positioned over the dorsal surface of the proximal tibia.

Procedure

1. The stabilizing hand holds the femur in position.
2. The manipulating hand glides the tibia in a ventral direction.

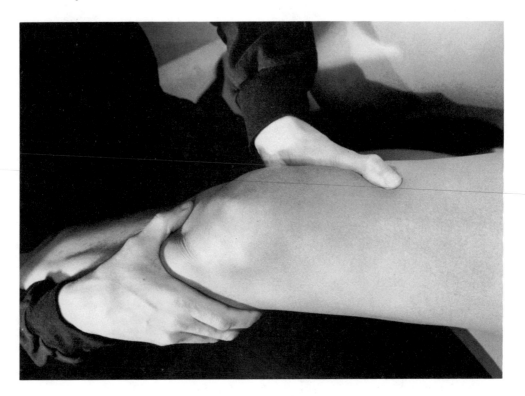

Medial Glide (Fig 6–7)

Purpose

- To increase joint play in the tibiofemoral joint
- To increase overall range of motion in the tibiofemoral joint
- To decrease pain in the knee
- To increase nutrition to articular structures

Positioning

1. The patient is either supine or sitting.
2. The tibiofemoral joint is positioned in the resting position if conservative techniques are indicated or approximating the restricted range if more aggressive techniques are indicated.
3. The clinician is at the foot of the treatment table between the patient's knees with the patient's lower leg between the clinician's arm and trunk.
4. The stabilizing hand grips the distal femur from the medial side.
5. The manipulating hand grips the proximal tibia and fibula from the lateral side.

Procedure

1. The stabilizing hand holds the femur in position.
2. The manipulating hand glides the proximal tibia in a medial direction indirectly through the fibula while the trunk guides the motion.

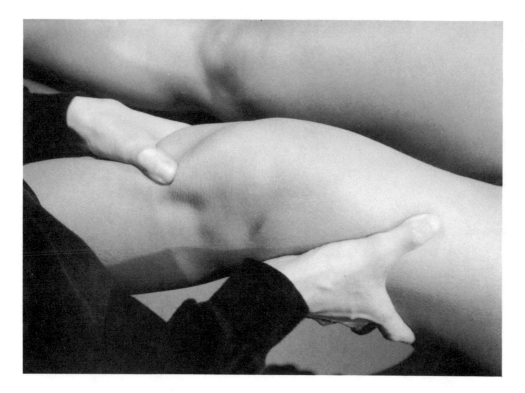

Lateral Glide (Fig 6–8)

Purpose

- To increase joint play in the tibiofemoral joint
- To increase overall range of motion in the tibiofemoral joint
- To decrease pain in the knee
- To increase nutrition to articular structures

Positioning

1. The patient is either supine or sitting.
2. The tibiofemoral joint is positioned in the resting position if conservative techniques are indicated or approximating the restricted range if more aggressive techniques are indicated.
3. The clinician is at the foot of the treatment table facing the patient's knee with the patient's lower leg between the clinician's arm and trunk.
4. The stabilizing hand grips the distal femur from the lateral side.
5. The manipulating hand grips the proximal tibia from the medial side.

Procedure

1. The stabilizing hand holds the femur in position.
2. The manipulating hand glides the proximal tibia in a lateral direction while the trunk guides the motion.

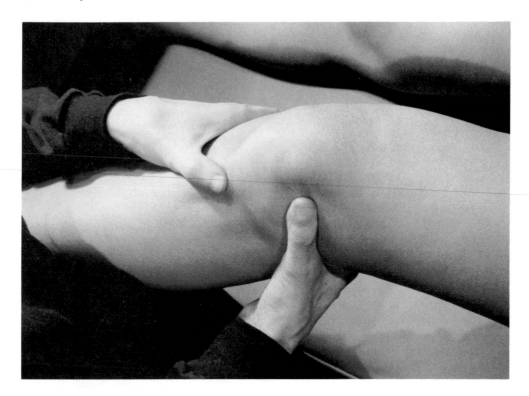

Medial Gap (Fig 6–9)

Purpose

- To increase joint play in the tibiofemoral joint
- To increase overall range of motion in the tibiofemoral joint
- To decrease pain in the knee
- To increase nutrition to articular structures

Positioning

1. The patient is either supine or sitting.
2. The tibiofemoral joint is positioned in the resting position if conservative techniques are indicated or approximating the restricted range if more aggressive techniques are indicated.
3. The clinician is at the foot of the treatment table facing the patient's knee with the patient's lower leg between the clinician's arm and trunk.
4. The stabilizing hand supports the distal lower leg from the medial side and holds the lower leg against the clinician's trunk.
5. The manipulating hand grips the lateral side of the knee at the joint line.

Procedure

1. The stabilizing hand holds the lower leg in position.
2. The manipulating hand moves the knee at the lateral joint line in a medial direction, thus creating a gapping at the joint line medially.

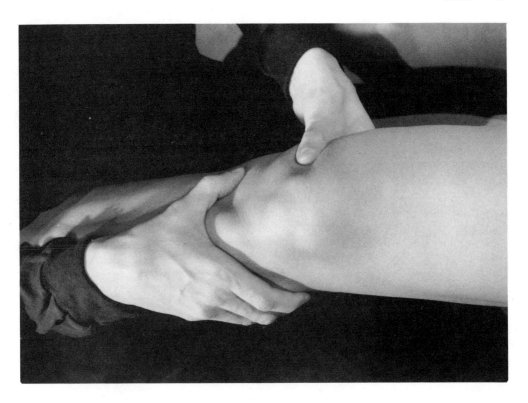

Lateral Gap (Fig 6–10)

Purpose

- To increase joint play in the tibiofemoral joint
- To increase overall range of motion in the tibiofemoral joint
- To decrease pain in the knee
- To increase nutrition to articular structures

Positioning

1. The patient is either supine or sitting.
2. The tibiofemoral joint is positioned in the resting position if conservative techniques are indicated or approximating the restricted range if more aggressive techniques are indicated.
3. The clinician is between the patient's knees with the patient's lower leg between the clinician's arm and trunk.
4. The stabilizing hand supports the distal lower leg from the lateral side and holds the lower leg against the clinician's trunk.
5. The manipulating hand grips the medial side of the knee at the joint line.

Procedure

1. The stabilizing hand holds the lower leg in position.
2. The manipulating hand moves the knee at the medial joint line in a lateral direction, thus creating a gapping at the joint line laterally.

Patellofemoral Joint

Osteokinematic degrees of freedom:	2 motions:
	Flexion/extension
	Medial/lateral glide
Ligaments:	Patellofemoral ligament
Joint orientation:	Patella: Dorsal
	Femur: Ventral
Type of joint:	Synovial
Joint surface anatomy:	Ovoid
	Patella: Convex
	Femur: Concave
Resting position:	Full extension
Close-packed position	Full flexion
Capsular pattern of restriction:	Flexion > extension

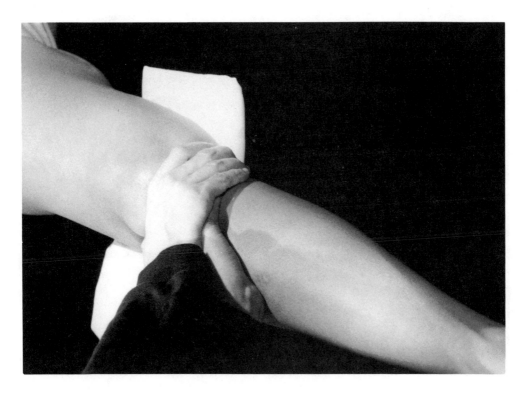

Cranial Glide (Fig 6–11)

Purpose

- To increase joint play in the patellofemoral joint
- To increase range of motion into knee extension
- To decrease pain in the knee
- To increase nutrition to articular structures

Positioning

1. The patient is supine.
2. The knee is positioned in slight flexion by placing a rolled towel underneath the knee.
3. The clinician is at the patient's lower leg facing the patellofemoral joint.
4. The manipulating hand is positioned with either the web space or the heel of the hand on the caudal surface of the patella.
5. The guiding hand is positioned over the manipulating hand.

Procedure

1. The manipulating hand glides the patella in a cranial direction.
2. The guiding hand controls the position of the manipulating hand.

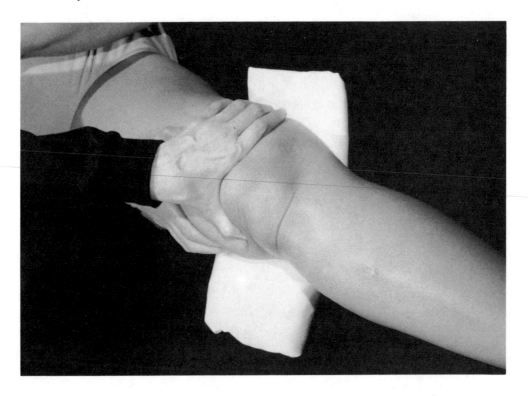

Caudal Glide (Fig 6–12)

Purpose

- To increase joint play in the patellofemoral joint
- To increase range of motion into knee flexion
- To decrease pain in the knee
- To increase nutrition to articular structures

Positioning

1. The patient is supine.
2. The knee is positioned in slight flexion by placing a rolled towel underneath the knee.
3. The clinician is at the patient's hip facing the patellofemoral joint.
4. The manipulating hand is positioned with either the web space or the heel of the hand on the cranial surface of the patella.
5. The guiding hand is positioned over the manipulating hand.

Procedure

1. The manipulating hand glides the patella in a caudal direction, taking care to avoid compressing the patella into the femur as much as possible by attempting to position the web space under the patella before initiating the technique.
2. The guiding hand controls the position of the manipulating hand.

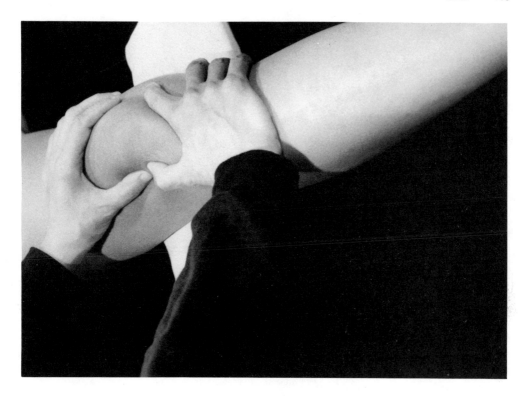

Medial Glide (Fig 6 – 13)

Purpose

- To increase joint play in the patellofemoral joint
- To increase range of motion into knee flexion
- To increase medial tracking of the patella with knee range of motion
- To decrease pain in the knee
- To increase nutrition to articular structures

Positioning

1. The patient is supine.
2. The knee is positioned in slight flexion by placing a rolled towel underneath the knee.
3. The clinician is at the patient's side facing the patellofemoral joint.
4. Both hands are positioned with either the thumb or the heel of the hand on the lateral surface of the patella.

Procedure

1. Both hands glide the patella in a medial direction.

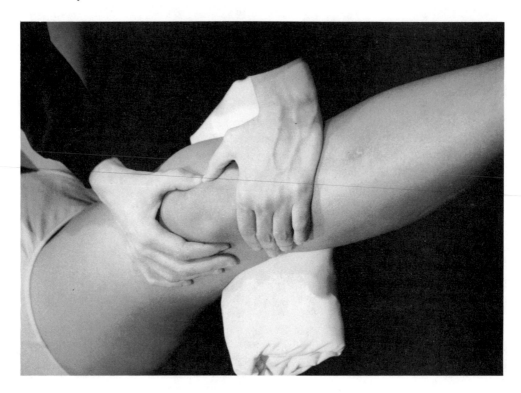

Lateral Glide (Fig 6–14)

Purpose

- To increase joint play in the patellofemoral joint
- To increase range of motion into knee flexion
- To increase lateral tracking of the patella with knee range of motion
- To decrease pain in the knee
- To increase nutrition to articular structures

Positioning

1. The patient is supine.
2. The knee is positioned in slight flexion by placing a rolled towel underneath the knee.
3. The clinician is at the patient's side facing the patellofemoral joint.
4. Both hands are positioned with either the thumb or the heel of the hand on the medial surface of the patella.

Procedure

1. Both hands glide the patella in a lateral direction.

REFERENCES

1. Hehne HJ: Biomechanics of the patellofemoral joint and its clinical relevance. *Clin Orthop* 1990; 258:73.
2. Hungerford DS, Barry M: Biomechanics of the patellofemoral joint. *Clin Orthop* 1979; 144:9.
3. Kettelkamp DB: Clinical implications of knee biomechanics. *Arch Surg* 1973; 107:406.
4. Laubenthal KN, Smidt GL, Kettelkamp DB: A quantitative analysis of knee motion during activities of daily living. *Phys Ther* 1972; 52:34.
5. Shapeero LG et al: Functional dynamics of the knee joint by Ultrafast, Cine-CT: *Invest Radiol* 1988; 23:118.

Figure 7 – 1

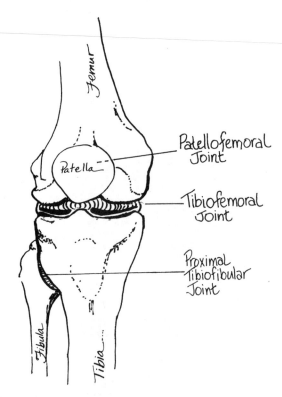

Proximal Tibiofibular Joint

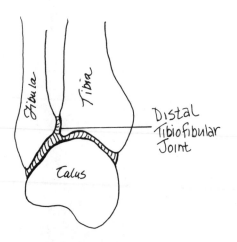

Distal Tibiofibular Joint

Chapter 7

Lower Leg

The lower leg consists of the proximal and distal tibiofibular joints. Motion at the tibiofibular joints corresponds primarily with motion at the foot, although a small degree of fibular ventral movement occurs with knee flexion.[3] Because the tibia and fibula are connected by the interosseus membrane, movement at the two joints is interrelated in a manner similar to that of the proximal and distal radioulnar joints of the forearm.

Positional faults are not uncommon at the proximal tibiofibular joint. A dorsal positional fault is especially common after an inversion injury of the ankle.

DORSIFLEXION AND PLANTAR FLEXION

With talocrural dorsiflexion the fibula glides cranially, and with plantar flexion it glides caudally.[2] The fibula also rotates laterally with dorsiflexion.[1] The talus is shaped so that it is wider ventrally than dorsally; thus with ankle dorsiflexion the tibia and fibula spread slightly to accommodate the shape of the talus. Distracting the distal tibiofibular joint therefore may help restore ankle dorsiflexion. Motion is so slight at both of these joints, however, that it is doubtful that either ankle or knee motion will improve significantly after manipulation to these joints. In addition, these joints are often hypermobile. A careful evaluation therefore should precede any manipulation of the tibiofibular joints.

Proximal Tibiofibular Joint

Osteokinematic degrees of freedom:	2 motions: Cranial/caudal glide Ventral/dorsal glide
Ligaments:	Posterior tibiofibular ligament Anterior tibiofibular ligament
Joint orientation:	Tibia: Lateral, dorsal, caudal Fibula: Medial, ventral, cranial
Type of joint:	Synovial
Articular surface anatomy:	Ovoid Tibia: Convex Fibula: Concave
Resting position:	25 degrees knee flexion, 10 degrees plantar flexion
Close-packed position:	None known
Capsular pattern of restriction:	None known

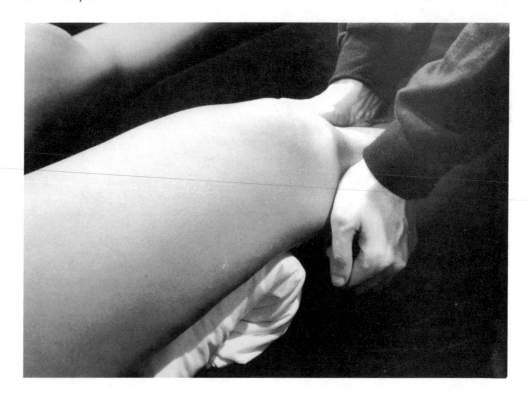

Dorsal Glide of Fibular Head (Fig 7–2)

Purpose

- To increase joint play in the proximal tibiofibular joint
- To reduce a ventral positional fault of the fibula
- To decrease pain in the upper lateral aspect of the lower leg
- To increase nutrition to articular structures

Positioning

1. The patient is supine with the knee supported by a pillow.
2. The proximal tibiofibular joint is positioned in the resting position.
3. The clinician is at the patient's side facing the knee.
4. The stabilizing hand grips the lower leg from the medial side.
5. The manipulating hand is positioned with the heel of the hand on the ventral surface of the fibular head.

Procedure

1. The stabilizing hand holds the lower leg in position.
2. The manipulating hand glides the proximal fibula in a dorsal direction.

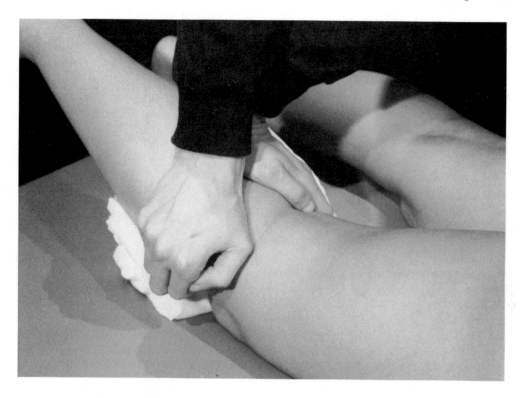

Ventral Glide of Fibular Head (Fig 7–3)

Purpose

- To increase joint play in the proximal tibiofibular joint
- To reduce a dorsal positional fault of the fibula
- To decrease pain in the upper lateral aspect of the lower leg
- To increase nutrition to articular structures

Positioning

1. The patient is prone with the foot supported by a pillow.
2. The proximal tibiofibular joint is positioned in the resting position.
3. The clinician is at the patient's unaffected side facing the knee.
4. The stabilizing hand grips the lower leg from the medial side.
5. The manipulating hand is positioned with the heel of the hand on the dorsal surface of the fibular head.

Procedure

1. The stabilizing hand holds the lower leg in position.
2. The manipulating hand glides the proximal fibula in a ventral direction.

Distal Tibiofibular Joint

Osteokinematic degrees of freedom:	2 motions:
	    Cranial/caudal glide
	    Ventral/dorsal glide

Ligaments:	Anterior tibiofibular ligament Posterior tibiofibular ligament Inferior transverse ligament Interosseous membrane
Joint orientation:	Tibia: Lateral Fibula: Medial
Type of joint:	Syndesmosis
Joint surface anatomy:	Ovoid Tibia: Concave Fibula: Convex
Resting position:	10 degrees plantarflexion, 5 degrees inversion
Close-packed position:	None; not a synovial joint
Capsular pattern of restriction:	None; not a synovial joint

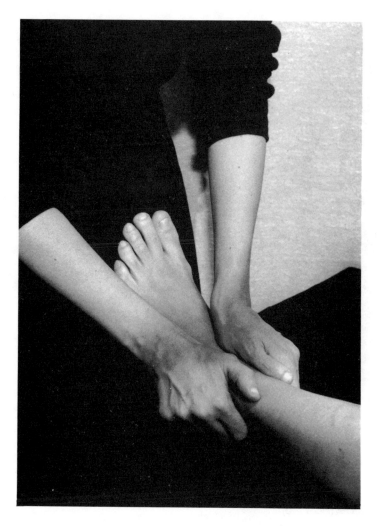

Distraction: Spreading Manipulation (Fig 7–4)

Purpose

- To increase joint play in the distal tibiofibular joint
- To increase range of motion into ankle dorsiflexion
- To decrease pain in the lower leg

Positioning

1. The patient is supine.
2. The joint is in the resting position.
3. The clinician is at the foot of the treatment table facing the patient's lower leg.
4. Both hands are positioned on the distal lower leg, one hand grips the fibula on the lateral surface, and the other hand grips the tibia on the medial surface.

Procedure

1. Both hands move the tibia and fibula away from each other.

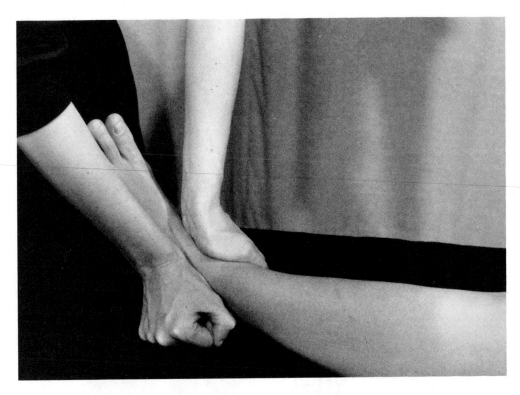

Dorsal Glide (Fig 7–5)

Purpose

- To increase joint play in the distal tibiofibular joint
- To increase range of motion into ankle plantarflexion
- To decrease pain in the lower lateral aspect of the lower leg

Positioning

1. The patient is supine.
2. The joint is in the resting position.
3. The clinician is at the foot of the treatment table facing the patient's lower leg.
4. The stabilizing hand grips the distal tibia.
5. The manipulating hand is positioned with the heel of the hand over the ventral surface of the lateral malleolus.

Procedure

1. The stabilizing hand holds the tibia in position.
2. The manipulating hand glides the lateral malleolus in a dorsal direction.

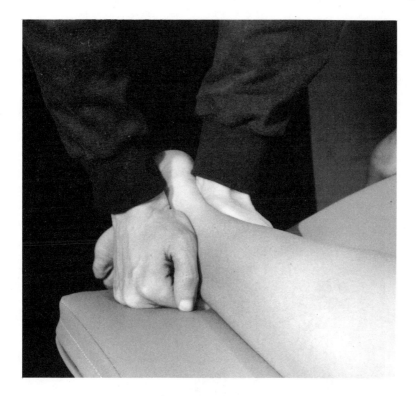

Ventral Glide (Fig 7–6)

Purpose

- To increase joint play in the distal tibiofibular joint
- To increase range of motion into ankle dorsiflexion
- To decrease pain in the lower lateral aspect of the lower leg

Positioning

1. The patient is prone.
2. The joint is in the resting position.
3. The clinician is at the foot of the treatment table facing the patient's lower leg.
4. The stabilizing hand grips the distal tibia.
5. The manipulating hand is positioned with the heel of the hand over the dorsal surface of the lateral malleolus.

Procedure

1. The stabilizing hand holds the tibia in position.
2. The manipulating hand glides the lateral malleolus in a ventral direction.

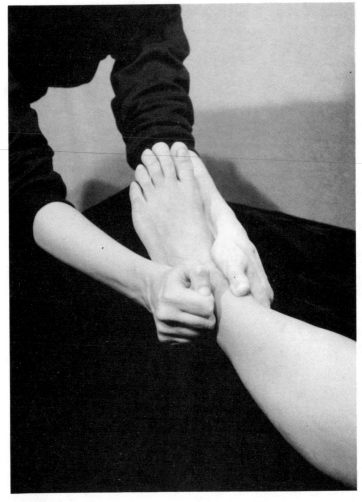

Cranial Glide (Fig 7—7)

Purpose

- To increase joint play in the distal tibiofibular joint
- To increase range of motion into ankle dorsiflexion
- To decrease pain in the lower lateral aspect of the lower leg

Positioning

1. The patient is supine.
2. The joint is in the resting position.
3. The clinician is at the foot of the treatment table facing the patient's lower leg.
4. The stabilizing hand grips the distal tibia.
5. The manipulating hand is positioned with the heel of the hand over the distal aspect of the lateral malleolus.

Procedure

1. The stabilizing hand holds the tibia in position.
2. The manipulating hand glides the fibular shaft in a cranial direction.

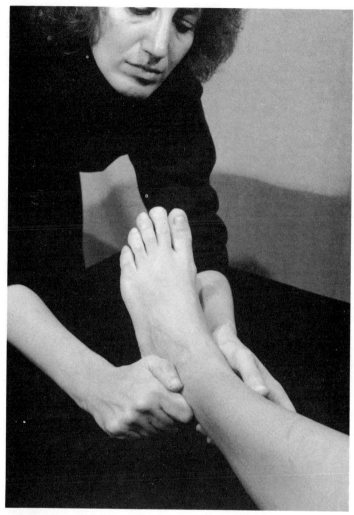

Caudal Glide (Fig 7–8)

Purpose

- To increase joint play in the distal tibiofibular joint
- To increase range of motion into ankle plantarflexion
- To decrease pain in the lower lateral aspect of the lower leg

Positioning

1. The patient is supine.
2. The joint is in the resting position.
3. The clinician is at the foot of the treatment table facing the patient's lower leg.
4. The stabilizing hand grips the distal tibia.
5. The manipulating hand grips the fibula by hooking the index finger around the cranial surface of the lateral malleolus.

Procedure

1. The stabilizing hand holds the tibia in position.
2. The manipulating hand glides the fibular shaft in a caudal direction.

REFERENCES

1. Barnett CH, Napier JR: The axis of rotation of the ankle joint in man. Its influence upon the form of the talus and the mobility of the fibula. *J Anat* 1952; 86:1.
2. Lapidus PW: Kinesiology and mechanical anatomy of the tarsal joints. *Clin Orthop* 1963; 30:20.
3. Ogden JA: The anatomy and function of the proximal tibiofibular joint. *Clin Orthop* 1974; 101:186.

Figure 8 – 1

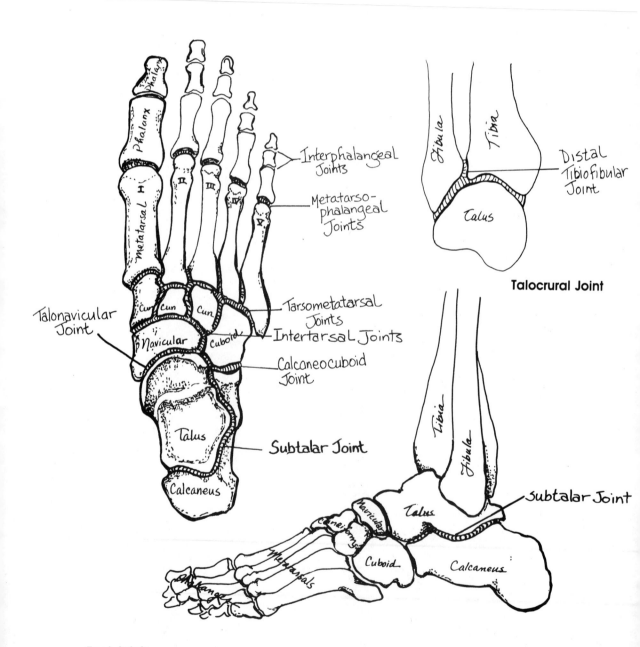

Interphalangeal Joints

Metatarso-phalangeal Joints

Talonavicular Joint

Tarsometatarsal Joints

Intertarsal Joints

Calcaneocuboid Joint

Subtalar Joint

Distal Tibiofibular Joint

Talocrural Joint

Subtalar Joint

Foot Joints

Chapter 8

Ankle and Foot

Ankle and foot motion most commonly is described as triplanar. The combined motion of dorsiflexion, abduction, and eversion, and plantar flexion, adduction, and inversion occur together but to a different extent at each of the following five joints in the ankle and foot: the talocrural joint, the subtalar joint, the midtarsal joint, the first ray, and the fifth ray.[8] These composite motions are called pronation and supination, respectively. Range of motion is considered functional if 10 to 20 degrees of dorsiflexion is present, 20 to 30 degrees of plantar flexion is present, and there is 6 to 10 degrees of motion equally divided between pronation and supination.[2]

Although triplanar motion is present at all major joints in the ankle and foot, dorsiflexion and plantar flexion are the primary motions at the talocrural joint, and inversion and eversion at the subtalar joint. Dorsiflexion and plantar flexion predominate along the oblique axis, and inversion and eversion along the longitudinal axis of the midtarsal joint. At the more distal joints, dorsiflexion and plantar flexion are the primary motions, except at the intermetatarsal joint, which allows the transverse arch of the forefoot to increase and decrease. These movements at the ankle and foot allow for a flexible base of support that accommodates changes in tibial rotation and produces a smooth transition from supination to pronation and back to supination during the stance phase of gait.

DORSIFLEXION AND PLANTAR FLEXION

The talocrural joint consists of a convex talus on a concave tibia and fibula. Dorsiflexion and plantar flexion are restored by gliding the talus dorsally and ventrally, respectively. The talus is wider ventrally; therefore the tibia and fibula must spread slightly to permit full motion into dorsiflexion.[6, 10] This joint play motion is restored by distracting the ventral tibia from the fibula (see Chapter 7).

PRONATION AND SUPINATION

The subtalar joint consists of a dorsal concave talar facet articulating on a convex calcaneus, and a ventral and medial convex talar facet articulating on a concave calcaneus. Talocalcaneal motion can be characterized as rotational. During closed-chain pronation the talus rotates such that the ventral surface moves medially and the dorsal surface moves laterally.[4, 7] This often is described as talar adduction. The talus also plantar flexes during pronation. At the same time the calcaneus moves into a valgus position.[3, 5] The opposite occurs with supination. With open-chain motion the moving bone is the calcaneus. Joint play for subtalar eversion therefore can be restored by rotating the ventral calcaneus laterally while simultaneously tilting the calcaneus into valgus position; subtalar inversion can be restored by rotating the ventral calcaneus medially while simultaneously tilting the calcaneus into varus position.

The midtarsal joint consists of the talonavicular and calcaneocuboid articulations. Movement occurs around two axes, one located longitudinally and the other in an oblique orientation. To restore eversion along the longitudinal axis at the midtarsal joint the navicular must either glide in a plantar direction or spin so that the medial surface moves in a plantar direction on the talus. The navicular glides or spins in a dorsal or dorsolateral direction on the talus with dorsiflexion at the oblique axis. The opposite takes place at the talonavicular joint during inversion along the longitudinal axis and during plantar flexion along the oblique axis. This occurs because the talus is convex articulating on a concave navicular.

The calcaneocuboid joint is a sellar joint, consisting of a convex calcaneus articulating on a concave cuboid in the longitudinal axis and a concave calcaneus articulating on a convex cuboid in the oblique axis. The cuboid must either glide dorsally or spin so that the lateral surface moves in a dorsal direction on the calcaneus for eversion to occur in the longitudinal axis, and in a plantar or plantomedial direction for dorsiflexion to occur along the oblique axis. The opposite occurs with calcaneocuboid inversion and plantar flexion, respectively.

Great care must be taken when treating the midtarsal joints with manipulation techniques, because most often these joints are hypermobile. In general, the best strategy is to evaluate carefully joint play and to treat by restoring limited motions and stabilizing excessive mobility based on the evaluative findings rather than the corresponding range of motion.

Intercuneiform, tarsometatarsal, and intertarsal motion all contribute to foot motion and should also be assessed.

TOE FLEXION AND EXTENSION

Toe flexion and extension occur at the metatarsophalangeal and interphalangeal joints. All these joints are convex proximally and concave distally; therefore, oscillations to restore motion should occur in the direction of the restriction. Motion at the first metatarsophalangeal joint frequently is restricted. Approximately 65 to 70 degrees of extension is required at this joint for normal push-off during gait.[8] Slightly less than 65 degrees of extension is necessary for normal gait at the other metatarsophalangeal joints.[8] Motion at the first metatarsophalangeal joint consists primarily of gliding, with some rotational component,[9] and therefore responds well to oscillation techniques.

TOE ABDUCTION AND ADDUCTION

Toe abduction and adduction occur at the metatarsophalangeal joints of all the toes, and if restricted, can be restored by gliding in the direction of the restriction.

Talocrural Joint

Osteokinematic degrees of freedom:	2 motions:
	    Dorsiflexion/plantar flexion
	    Rotation

Ligaments:	Deltoid ligament (anterior tibiotalar, posterior tibiotalar, tibiocalcaneal, tibionavicular) Lateral collateral ligament (anterior talofibular, posterior talofibular, calcaneofibular)
Joint orientation:	Tibia: Caudal, lateral Fibula: Medial Talus: Cranial, medial, lateral
Type of joint:	Synovial

Articular surface anatomy:	Sellar
	Tibia and Fibula:
	    Concave ventral to dorsal (dorsiflexion/plantar flexion)
	    Convex medial to lateral (inversion/eversion)
	Talus:
	    Convex ventral to dorsal (dorsiflexion/plantar flexion)
	    Concave medial to lateral (inversion/eversion)

Resting position:	10 degrees plantar flexion and midway between inversion and eversion
Close-packed position:	Full dorsiflexion
Capsular pattern of restriction:	Plantar flexion > dorsiflexion

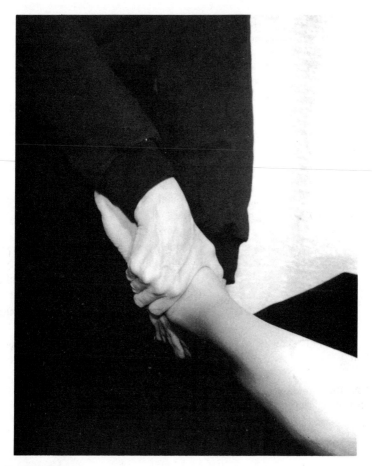

Distraction (Fig 8–2)

Purpose

- To increase joint play in the talocrural joint
- To increase overall range of motion in the talocrural joint
- To decrease pain in the ankle
- To increase nutrition to articular structures

Positioning

1. The patient is supine.
2. The talocrural joint is positioned in the resting position if conservative techniques are indicated or approximating the restricted range if more aggressive techniques are indicated.
3. The clinician is at the foot of the table facing the plantar surface of the patient's foot.
4. Both hands grip the proximal talus.
5. The clinician's arms are lined up with the patient's leg.

Procedure

1. Both hands move the talus distally as the clinician leans away from the joint.

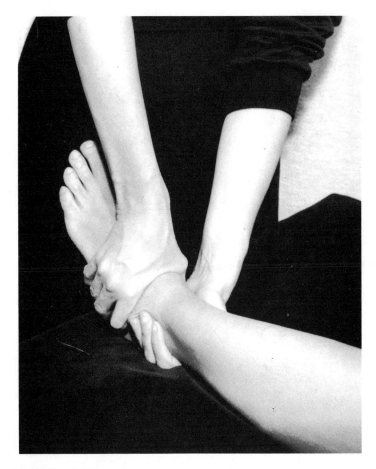

Dorsal Glide (Fig 8–3)

Purpose

- To increase joint play in the talocrural joint
- To increase range of motion into ankle dorsiflexion
- To decrease pain in the ankle
- To increase nutrition to articular structures

Positioning

1. The patient is supine.
2. The talocrural joint is positioned in the resting position if conservative techniques are indicated or approximating the restricted range if more aggressive techniques are indicated.
3. The clinician is at the foot of the table facing the plantar surface of the patient's foot.
4. The manipulating hand grips talus at the ventral surface of the lower leg with the web space.
5. The stabilizing hand is positioned on the dorsal surface of the distal lower leg.

Procedure

1. The manipulating hand glides the talus in a dorsal direction.
2. The stabilizing hand holds the lower leg in position.

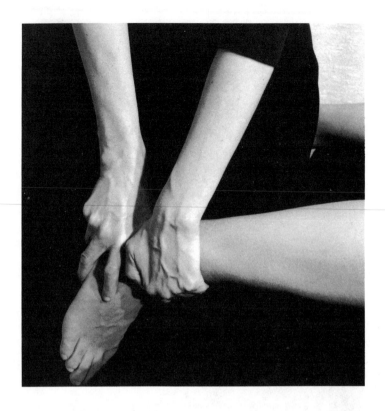

Ventral Glide: First Technique (Fig 8–4)

Purpose

- To increase joint play in the talocrural joint
- To increase range of motion into ankle plantar flexion
- To decrease pain in the ankle
- To increase nutrition to articular structures

Positioning

1. The patient is prone.
2. The talocrural joint is positioned in the resting position if conservative techniques are indicated or approximating the restricted range if more aggressive techniques are indicated.
3. The clinician is at the foot of the table facing the plantar surface of the patient's foot.
4. The stabilizing hand is positioned on the ventral surface of the lower leg.
5. The manipulating hand grips the talus at the dorsal surface of the lower leg if the ankle is in the resting position, or the calcaneus at the dorsal surface of the lower leg if the foot is in too much plantarflexion to permit contact with the talus.

Procedure

1. The stabilizing hand holds the lower leg in position.
2. The manipulating hand glides the talus in a ventral direction either directly or through the calcaneus.

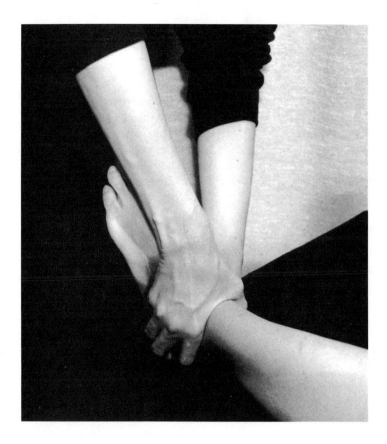

Ventral Glide: Second Technique (Fig 8–5)

Purpose

- To increase joint play in the talocrural joint
- To increase range of motion into ankle plantar flexion
- To decrease pain in the ankle
- To increase nutrition to articular structures

Positioning

1. The patient is supine.
2. The talocrural joint is positioned in the resting position if conservative techniques are indicated or approximating the restricted range if more aggressive techniques are indicated.
3. The clinician is at the foot of the table facing the plantar surface of the patient's foot.
4. The stabilizing hand grips the talus on the dorsal surface of the lower leg.
5. The manipulating hand grips the distal tibia and fibula at the ventral surface of the lower leg.

Procedure

1. The stabilizing hand holds the talus in position.
2. The manipulating hand glides the tibia and fibula in a dorsal direction, thus imparting a ventral force to the talus on the tibia and fibula.

Subtalar Joint

Osteokinematic degrees of freedom:	1 motion: Inversion/eversion
Ligaments:	Interosseous talocalcaneal ligament Cervical ligament Lateral talocalcaneal ligament Medial talocalcaneal ligament
Joint orientation:	Talus: Caudal, dorsal, lateral Calcaneus: Cranial, ventral, medial
Type of joint:	Synovial

Articular surface anatomy:	Ovoid
	Talar facets:
	    Dorsal facet, concave
	    Two ventral facets, convex
	Calcaneal facets:
	    Dorsal facet, convex
	    Two ventral facets, concave

Resting position:	Midway between inversion and eversion with 10 degrees of plantarflexion
Close-packed position:	Full inversion
Capsular pattern of restriction:	Inversion > eversion

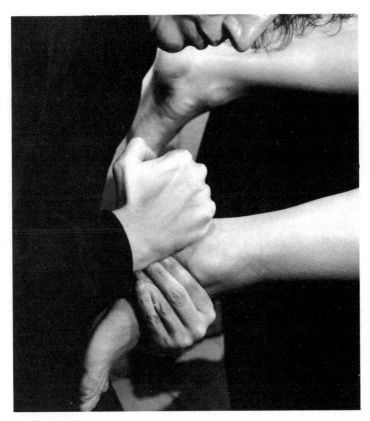

Distraction (Fig 8–6)

Purpose

- To increase joint play in the subtalar joint
- To increase overall range of motion in the subtalar joint
- To decrease pain in the ankle
- To increase nutrition to articular structures

Positioning

1. The patient is prone with the foot off the table.
2. The subtalar joint is positioned in the resting position if conservative techniques are indicated or approximating the restricted range if more aggressive techniques are indicated.
3. The clinician is at the foot of the table facing the plantar surface of the patient's foot.
4. The stabilizing hand grips the talus at the ventral surface of the lower leg with the web space.
5. The manipulating hand grips the calcaneus at the dorsal surface of the lower leg with the ulnar border of the hand.

Procedure

1. The stabilizing hand holds the talus in position and controls the position of the foot.
2. The manipulating hand moves the calcaneus distally.

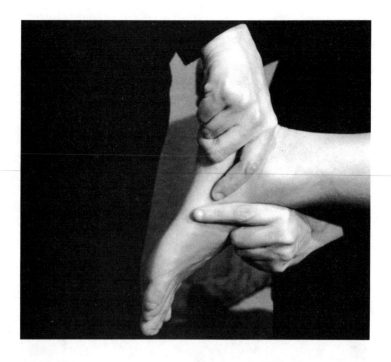

Eversion Manipulation (Fig 8–7)

Purpose

- To increase joint play in the subtalar joint
- To increase range of motion into subtalar eversion
- To decrease pain in the ankle
- To increase nutrition to articular structures

Positioning

1. The patient is prone with the foot off the table.
2. The subtalar joint is positioned in the resting position if conservative techniques are indicated or approximating the restricted range if more aggressive techniques are indicated.
3. The clinician is at the foot of the table facing the plantar aspect of the patient's foot.
4. The stabilizing hand grips the talus at the ventral surface of the lower leg with the web space.
5. The manipulating hand grips the calcaneus at the dorsal surface of the lower leg with the web space.

Procedure

1. The stabilizing hand holds the talus in position.
2. The manipulating hand glides the calcaneus in a rotational direction by pushing the ventromedial calcaneus laterally and the dorsolateral calcaneus medially while simultaneously gliding the calcaneus in a valgus direction.

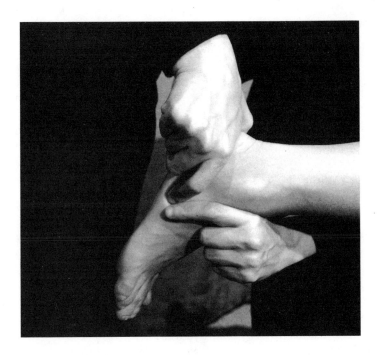

Inversion Manipulation (Fig 8–8)

Purpose

- To increase joint play in the subtalar joint
- To increase range of motion into subtalar inversion
- To decrease pain in the ankle
- To increase nutrition to articular structures

Positioning

1. The patient is prone with the foot off the table.
2. The subtalar joint is positioned in the resting position if conservative techniques are indicated or approximating the restricted range if more aggressive techniques are indicated.
3. The clinician is at the foot of the table facing the plantar aspect of the patient's foot.
4. The stabilizing hand grips the talus at the ventral surface of the lower leg with the web space.
5. The manipulating hand grips the calcaneus at the dorsal surface of the lower leg with the web space.

Procedure

1. The stabilizing hand holds the talus in position.
2. The manipulating hand glides the calcaneus in a rotational direction by pushing the dorsomedial calcaneus laterally and the ventrolateral calcaneus medially while simultaneously gliding the calcaneus in a varus direction.

Midtarsal Joints: Talonavicular and Calcaneocuboid

Osteokinematic degrees of freedom:	3 motions: The midtarsal joint consists of two joints, each of which has the same two axes, one that runs obliquely and one that runs longitudinally Oblique axis: 1 degree of freedom, dorsiflexion/plantarflexion Longitudinal axis: 1 degree of freedom, eversion/inversion
Ligaments:	Long plantar ligament Plantar calcaneonavicular ligament Bifurcate ligament
Joint orientation:	Talonavicular joint Talus: distal, lateral, dorsal Navicular: Proximal, medial, volar Calcaneocuboid joint Calcaneus: Distal, medial, dorsal Cuboid: Proximal, lateral, volar
Type of joint:	Synovial

Articular surface anatomy:	Talonavicular joint: Ovoid
	Talus: Convex
	Navicular: Concave
	Calcaneocuboid joint: Sellar
	Calcaneus:
	  Concave dorsal to plantar (oblique axis)
	  Convex proximal to distal (longitudinal axis)
	Cuboid:
	  Convex dorsal to plantar (oblique axis)
	  Concave proximal to distal (longitudinal axis)

Resting position:	Midway between supination and pronation with 10 degrees of plantarflexion
Close-packed position:	Full supination
Capsular pattern of restriction:	Supination > pronation

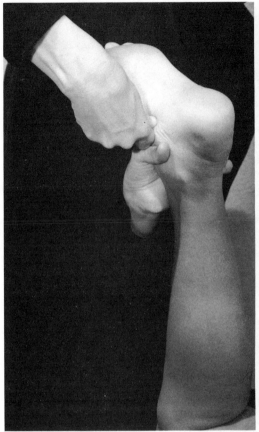 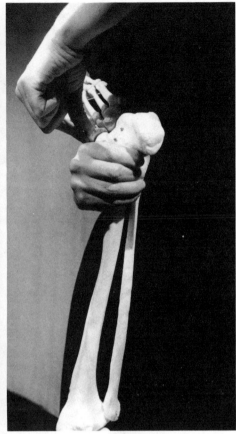

Navicular Dorsal Glide (Figs 8–9, 8–10)

Purpose

- To increase joint play in the talonavicular joint
- To increase range of motion into midtarsal inversion along the longitudinal axis
- To increase range of motion into midtarsal dorsiflexion along the oblique axis
- To decrease pain in the foot
- To increase nutrition to articular structures

Positioning

1. The patient is prone with the knee flexed to 90 degrees.
2. The joint is in the resting position.
3. The clinician is facing the lateral aspect of the patient's foot.
4. The stabilizing hand grips the neck of the talus at the dorsal surface of the foot with the web space.
5. The manipulating hand is positioned on the navicular with the thumb on the plantar surface and the index finger on the dorsal surface.

Procedure

1. The stabilizing hand holds the talus in position.
2. The manipulating hand glides the navicular in a dorsal direction.

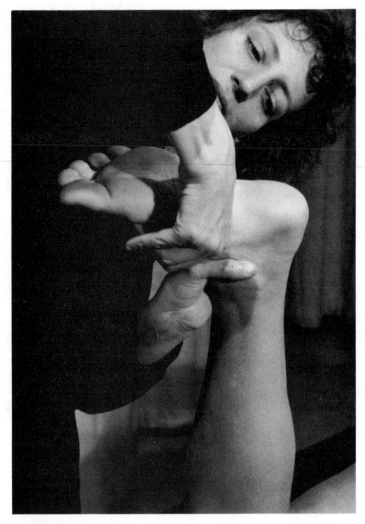

Navicular Dorsolateral Glide (Fig 8–11)

Purpose

- To increase joint play in the talonavicular joint
- To increase range of motion into midtarsal inversion along the longitudinal axis
- To increase range of motion into midtarsal dorsiflexion along the oblique axis
- To decrease pain in the foot
- To increase nutrition to articular structures

Positioning

1. The patient is prone with the knee flexed to 90 degrees.
2. The joint is in the resting position.
3. The clinician is facing the lateral aspect of the patient's foot.
4. The stabilizing hand grips the neck of the talus at the dorsal surface of the foot with the web space.
5. The manipulating hand is positioned with the web space over the plantar surface of the navicular.

Procedure

1. The stabilizing hand holds the talus in position.
2. The manipulating hand glides the medial navicular in a dorsolateral direction, thus rotating the navicular into a more supinated position.

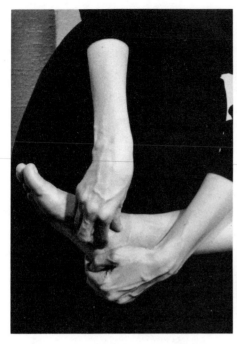
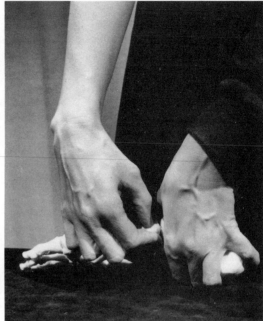

Navicular Plantar Glide (Figs 8–12, 8–13)

Purpose

- To increase joint play in the talonavicular joint
- To increase range of motion into midtarsal eversion along the longitudinal axis
- To increase range of motion into midtarsal plantarflexion along the oblique axis
- To decrease pain in the foot
- To increase nutrition to articular structures

Positioning

1. The patient is supine.
2. The joint is in the resting position.
3. The clinician is facing the lateral aspect of the patient's foot.
4. The stabilizing hand grips the neck of the talus at the plantar surface of the foot with the fingers.
5. Additional stabilization can be achieved by holding the patient's foot against the clinician's trunk.
6. The manipulating hand is positioned on the navicular with the thumb on the dorsal surface and the index finger on the plantar surface.

Procedure

1. The stabilizing hand holds the talus in position.
2. The manipulating hand glides the navicular in a plantar direction.

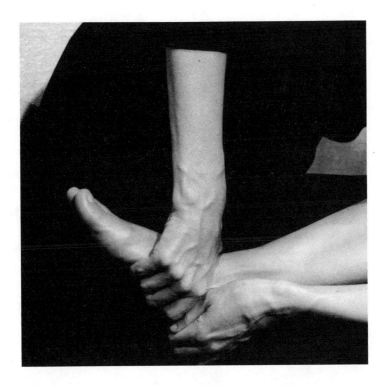

Navicular Plantarmedial Glide: Longitudinal Axis (Fig 8–14)

Purpose

- To increase joint play in the talonavicular joint
- To increase range of motion into midtarsal eversion along the longitudinal axis
- To increase range of motion into midtarsal plantarflexion along the oblique axis
- To decrease pain in the foot
- To increase nutrition to articular structures

Positioning

1. The patient is supine.
2. The joint is in the resting position.
3. The clinician is facing the lateral aspect of the patient's foot.
4. The stabilizing hand grips the neck of the talus at the plantar surface of the foot with the fingers.
5. Additional stabilization can be achieved by holding the patient's foot against the clinician's trunk.
6. The manipulating hand is positioned with the web space over the dorsal surface of the navicular.

Procedure

1. The stabilizing hand holds the talus in position.
2. The manipulating hand glides the medial navicular in a plantomedial direction, thus rotating the navicular into a more pronated position.

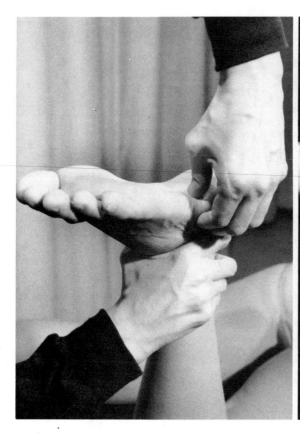 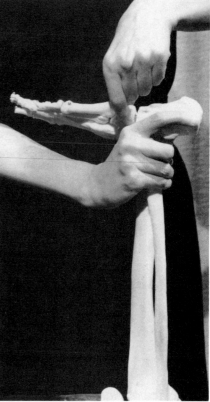

Cuboid Dorsal Glide (Figs 8–15, 8–16)

Purpose

- To increase joint play in the calcaneocuboid joint
- To increase range of motion into midtarsal eversion along the longitudinal axis
- To increase range of motion into midtarsal plantarflexion along the oblique axis
- To decrease pain in the foot
- To increase nutrition to articular structures

Positioning

1. The patient is prone with the knee flexed to 90 degrees.
2. The joint is in the resting position.
3. The clinician is facing the medial aspect of the patient's foot.
4. The stabilizing hand grips the calcaneus at the dorsal surface of the foot with the web space.
5. The manipulating hand is positioned on the cuboid with the thumb on the plantar surface and the index finger on the dorsal surface.

Procedure

1. The stabilizing hand holds the calcaneus in position.
2. The manipulating hand glides the cuboid in a dorsal direction.

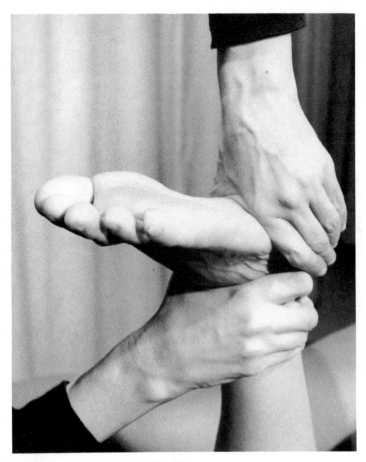

Cuboid Dorsolateral Glide (Fig 8–17)

Purpose

- To increase joint play in the calcaneocuboid joint
- To increase range of motion into midtarsal eversion along the longitudinal axis
- To increase range of motion into midtarsal plantarflexion along the oblique axis
- To decrease pain in the foot
- To increase nutrition to articular structures

Positioning

1. The patient is prone with the knee flexed to 90 degrees.
2. The joint is in the resting position.
3. The clinician is facing the medial aspect of the patient's foot.
4. The stabilizing hand grips the calcaneus at the dorsal surface of the foot with the web space.
5. The manipulating hand is positioned with the web space over the plantar surface of the cuboid.

Procedure

1. The stabilizing hand holds the calcaneus in position.
2. The manipulating hand glides the lateral cuboid in a dorsolateral direction, thus rotating the cuboid into a more pronated position.

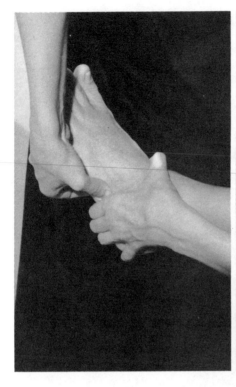 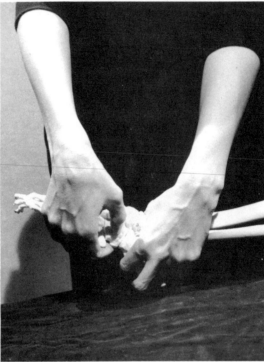

Cuboid Plantar Glide (Figs 8–18, 8–19)

Purpose

- To increase joint play in the calcaneocuboid joint
- To increase range of motion into midtarsal inversion along the longitudinal axis
- To increase range of motion into midtarsal dorsiflexion along the oblique axis
- To decrease pain in the foot
- To increase nutrition to articular structures

Positioning

1. The patient is supine.
2. The joint is in the resting position.
3. The clinician is facing the medial aspect of the patient's foot.
4. The stabilizing hand grips the calcaneus at the plantar surface of the foot with the fingers.
5. Additional stabilization can be achieved by holding the patient's foot against the clinician's trunk.
6. The manipulating hand is positioned on the cuboid with the thumb on the dorsal surface and the index finger on the plantar surface.

Procedure

1. The stabilizing hand holds the calcaneus in position.
2. The manipulating hand glides the cuboid in a plantar direction.

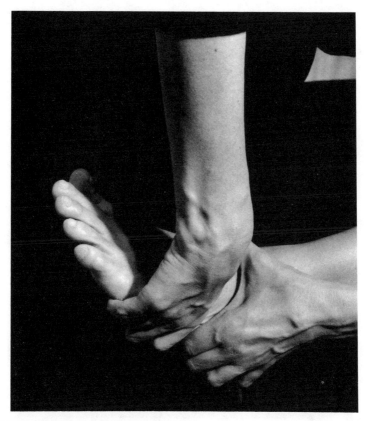

Cuboid Plantarmedial Glide (Fig 8–20)

Purpose

- To increase joint play in the calcaneocuboid joint
- To increase range of motion into midtarsal inversion along the longitudinal axis
- To increase range of motion into midtarsal dorsiflexion along the oblique axis
- To reduce a dorsolateral positional fault of the cuboid
- To decrease pain in the foot
- To increase nutrition to articular structures

Positioning

1. The patient is supine.
2. The joint is in the resting position.
3. The clinician is facing the medial aspect of the patient's foot.
4. The stabilizing hand grips the calcaneus at the plantar surface of the foot with the fingers.
5. Additional stabilization can be achieved by holding the patient's foot against the clinician's trunk.
6. The manipulating hand is positioned with the web space over the dorsal surface of the cuboid.

Procedure

1. The stabilizing hand holds the calcaneus in position.
2. The manipulating hand glides the lateral cuboid in a plantomedial direction, thus rotating the cuboid into a more supinated position.

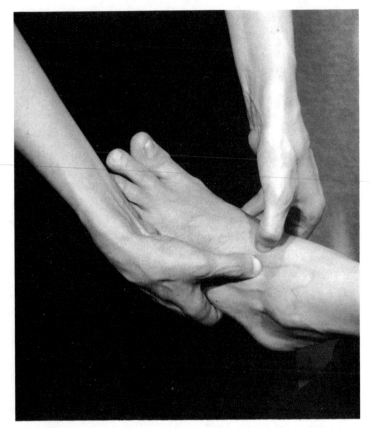

Specific Midtarsal Manipulations (Fig 8–21)

Purpose

- To increase joint play in the midtarsal joints
- To increase overall range of motion in the intertarsal joints
- To decrease pain in the foot
- To increase nutrition to articular structures

Positioning

1. The patient is supine.
2. The joint is in the resting position.
3. The clinician is facing the dorsal aspect of the foot.
4. Additional stabilization can be achieved by holding the patient's foot against the clinician's trunk.
5. The stabilizing hand grips the one tarsal bone with the thumb on the dorsal surface of the foot and the index finger on the plantar surface of the foot.
6. The manipulating hand grips the other tarsal bone with the thumb on the dorsal surface of the foot and the index finger on the plantar surface of the foot.

Procedure

1. The stabilizing hand holds the one tarsal bone in position.
2. The manipulating hand glides the cuboid in a dorsal direction on the navicular, the

cuboid in a plantar direction on the navicular, all cuneiforms in a dorsal direction on the navicular, all cuneiforms in a plantar direction on the navicular, the cuboid in a dorsal direction on the third cuneiform, and the cuboid in a plantar direction on the third cuneiform.

Tarsometatarsal Joints

Osteokinematic degrees of freedom:	1 motion:
	Dorsiflexion/plantarflexion
Ligaments:	Dorsal tarsometatarsal ligament
	Plantar tarsometatarsal ligament
Joint orientation:	First cuneiform: Distal, medial
	Second cuneiform: Distal, medial
	Third cuneiform: Distal
	Cuboid: Distal, lateral
	First and second metatarsal: Proximal, lateral
	Third metatarsal: Proximal
	Fourth and fifth metatarsal: Proximal, medial
Type of joint:	Synovial
Joint surface anatomy:	Ovoid
	Tarsals: Convex
	Metatarsals: Concave
Resting position:	Midway between supination and pronation
Close-packed position:	Full supination
Capsular pattern of restriction:	Not described

Dorsal Glide

Purpose

- To increase joint play in the tarsometatarsal joints
- To increase range of motion into dorsiflexion
- To decrease pain in the midfoot
- To increase nutrition to articular structures

Positioning

1. The patient is supine.
2. The joint is in the resting position.
3. The clinician is facing the dorsal surface of the foot.
4. The stabilizing hand grips the tarsal bone with the thumb on the dorsal surface of the foot and the index finger on the plantar surface of the foot.
5. Additional stabilization can be achieved by holding the patient's foot against the clinician's trunk.
6. The manipulating hand grips the metatarsal with the thumb on the dorsal surface of the foot and the index finger on the plantar surface of the foot.

Procedure

1. The stabilizing hand holds the tarsal bone in position.
2. The manipulating hand glides the first metatarsal in a dorsal direction on the first cuneiform, the second metatarsal in a dorsal direction on the second cuneiform, the

third metatarsal in a dorsal direction on the third cuneiform, the fourth metatarsal in a dorsal direction on the cuboid, and the fifth metatarsal in a dorsal direction on the cuboid.
3. Movement in these joints is minimal.

Plantar Glide

Purpose

- To increase joint play in the tarsometatarsal joints
- To increase range of motion into plantarflexion
- To decrease pain in the midfoot
- To increase nutrition to articular structures

Positioning

1. The patient is supine.
2. The joint is in the resting position.
3. The clinician is facing the dorsal surface of the foot.
4. The stabilizing hand grips the tarsal bone with the thumb on the dorsal surface of the foot and the index finger on the plantar surface of the foot.
5. Additional stabilization can be achieved by holding the patient's foot against the clinician's trunk.
6. The manipulating hand grips the metatarsal with the thumb on the dorsal surface of the foot and the index finger on the plantar surface of the foot.

Procedure

1. The stabilizing hand holds the tarsal bone in position.
2. The manipulating hand glides the first metatarsal in a plantar direction on the first cuneiform, the second metatarsal in a plantar direction on the second cuneiform, the third metatarsal in a plantar direction on the third cuneiform, the fourth metatarsal in a plantar direction on the cuboid, and the fifth metatarsal in a plantar direction on the cuboid.
3. Movement in these joints is minimal.

Intermetatarsal Joints

Osteokinematic degrees of freedom:	1 motion: Dorsal/plantar glide
Ligaments:	Transverse metatarsal ligament
Joint orientation:	Medial metatarsal: Lateral Lateral metatarsal: Medial
Type of joint:	Synarthrosis
Articular surface anatomy:	Ovoid, plane Metatarsal II, III, and IV lateral border: Convex Metatarsal I lateral border, metatarsal III, IV, and V medial border: Concave
Resting position:	Not described
Close-packed position:	None; not a synovial joint
Capsular pattern of restriction:	None; not a synovial joint

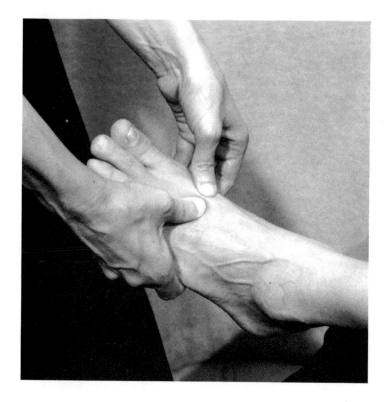

Dorsal Glide (Fig 8−22)

Purpose

- To increase joint play in the intermetatarsal articulations
- To increase range of motion into decreasing the transverse arch of the foot
- To decrease pain in the forefoot

Positioning

1. The patient is supine.
2. The foot is in a neutral position.
3. The clinician is facing the dorsal surface of the foot.
4. The stabilizing hand grips the midshaft of the one metatarsal with the thumb on the dorsal surface of the foot and the index finger on the plantar surface of the foot.
5. The manipulating hand grips the midshaft of the other metatarsal with the thumb on the dorsal surface of the foot and the index finger on the plantar surface of the foot.

Procedure

1. The stabilizing hand holds the one metatarsal in position.
2. The manipulating hand glides the first metatarsal in a dorsal direction on the second metatarsal, the third metatarsal in a dorsal direction on the second metatarsal, the fourth metatarsal in a dorsal direction on the third metatarsal, and the fifth metatarsal in a dorsal direction on the fourth metatarsal.

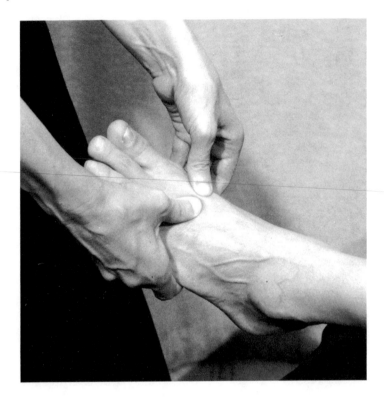

Plantar Glide (Fig 8–23)

Purpose

- To increase joint play in the intermetatarsal articulations
- To increase range of motion into increasing the transverse arch of the foot
- To decrease pain in the forefoot

Positioning

1. The patient is supine.
2. The foot is in a neutral position.
3. The clinician is facing the dorsal surface of the foot.
4. The stabilizing hand grips the midshaft of the one metatarsal with the thumb on the dorsal surface of the foot and the index finger on the plantar surface of the foot.
5. The manipulating hand grips the midshaft of the other metatarsal with the thumb on the dorsal surface of the foot and the index finger on the plantar surface of the foot.

Procedure

1. The stabilizing hand holds the one metatarsal in position.
2. The manipulating hand glides the first metatarsal in a plantar direction on the second metatarsal, the third metatarsal in a plantar direction on the second metatarsal, the fourth metatarsal in a plantar direction on the third metatarsal, and the fifth metatarsal in a plantar direction on the fourth metatarsal.

Metatarsophalangeal Joints

Osteokinematic degrees of freedom:	2 motions:
	    Flexion/extension
	    Abduction/adduction

Ligaments:	Plantar ligaments Collateral ligaments
Joint orientation:	Metatarsals: Distal Phalanges: Proximal
Type of joint:	Synovial
Articular surface anatomy:	Ovoid Metatarsals: Convex Phalanges: Concave
Resting position:	Midway between flexion and extension, and between abduction and adduction
Close-packed position:	Full extension
Capsular pattern of restriction:	First metatarsophalangeal joint: Extension > flexion Metatarsophalangeal joints 2 through 5: Flexion > extension

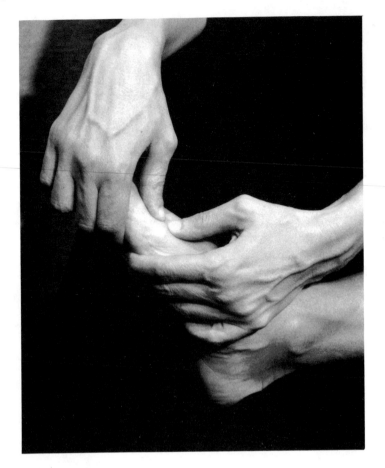

Distraction (Fig 8–24)

Purpose

- To increase joint play in the metatarsophalangeal joints
- To increase overall range of motion in the metatarsophalangeal joints
- To decrease pain in the toes
- To increase nutrition to articular structures

Positioning

1. The patient is supine.
2. The metatarsophalangeal joint is positioned in the resting position if conservative techniques are indicated or approximating the restricted range if more aggressive techniques are indicated.
3. The clinician is facing the dorsal surface of the foot.
4. The stabilizing hand grips the head of the metatarsal with the thumb on the dorsal surface of the foot and the index finger on the plantar surface of the foot.
5. The manipulating hand grips the proximal end of the proximal phalanx being manipulated with the thumb on the dorsal surface of the foot and the index finger on the plantar surface of the foot.

Procedure

1. The stabilizing hand holds the metatarsal in position.
2. The manipulating hand moves the base of the proximal phalanx distally.
3. The use of a padded tongue depressor may assist the clinician in directing a more precise manipulation.
4. The use of surgical gloves may allow the clinician to obtain a stronger grip by reducing slippage against the patient's skin.

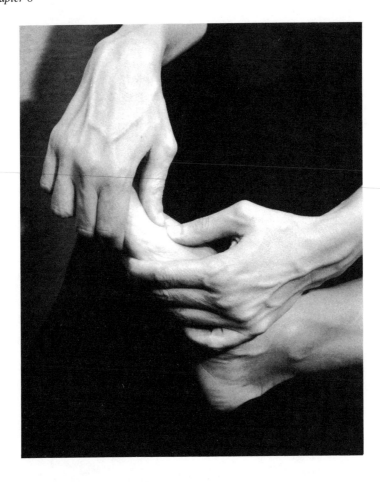

Dorsal Glide (Fig 8–25)

Purpose

- To increase joint play in the metatarsophalangeal joints
- To increase range of motion into metatarsophalangeal extension
- To decrease pain in the toes
- To increase nutrition to articular structures

Positioning

1. The patient is supine.
2. The metatarsophalangeal joint is positioned in the resting position if conservative techniques are indicated or approximating the restricted range if more aggressive techniques are indicated.
3. The clinician is facing the dorsal surface of the foot.
4. The stabilizing hand grips the head of the metatarsal with the thumb on the dorsal surface of the foot and the index finger on the plantar surface of the foot.
5. The manipulating hand grips the proximal end of the proximal phalanx being manipulated with the thumb on the dorsal surface of the foot and the index finger on the plantar surface of the foot.

Procedure

1. The stabilizing hand holds the metatarsal in position.
2. The manipulating hand glides the proximal phalanx in a dorsal direction.
3. The use of a padded tongue depressor may assist the clinician in directing a more precise manipulation.
4. The use of surgical gloves may allow the clinician to obtain a stronger grip by reducing slippage against the patient's skin.

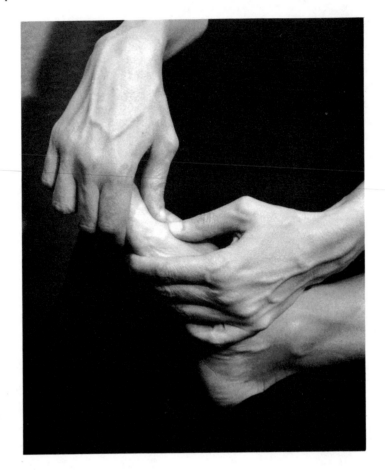

Plantar Glide (Fig 8–26)

Purpose

- To increase joint play in the metatarsophalangeal joints
- To increase range of motion into metatarsophalangeal flexion
- To decrease pain in the toes
- To increase nutrition to articular structures

Positioning

1. The patient is supine.
2. The metatarsophalangeal joint is positioned in the resting position if conservative techniques are indicated or approximating the restricted range if more aggressive techniques are indicated.
3. The clinician is facing the dorsal surface of the foot.
4. The stabilizing hand grips the head of the metatarsal with the thumb on the dorsal surface of the foot and the index finger on the plantar surface of the foot.
5. The manipulating hand grips the proximal end of the proximal phalanx being manipulated with the thumb on the dorsal surface of the foot and the index finger on the plantar surface of the foot.

Procedure

1. The stabilizing hand holds the metatarsal in position.
2. The manipulating hand glides the proximal phalanx in a plantar direction.
3. The use of a padded tongue depressor may assist the clinician in directing a more precise manipulation.
4. The use of surgical gloves may allow the clinician to obtain a stronger grip by reducing slippage against the patient's skin.

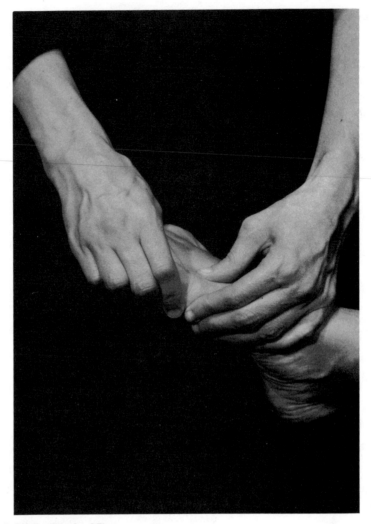

Medial Glide (Fig 8–27)

Purpose

- To increase joint play in the metatarsophalangeal joints
- To increase range of motion into metatarsophalangeal joint abduction of digits 1 and 2, tibial abduction of digit 3, and adduction of digits 4 and 5
- To decrease pain in the toes
- To increase nutrition to articular structures

Positioning

1. The patient is supine.
2. The metatarsophalangeal joint is positioned in the resting position if conservative techniques are indicated or approximating the restricted range if more aggressive techniques are indicated.
3. The clinician is facing the dorsal surface of the foot.
4. The stabilizing hand grips the head of the metatarsal with the thumb on the dorsal surface of the foot and the index finger on the plantar surface of the foot.

5. The manipulating hand grips the proximal end of the proximal phalanx being manipulated on the medial and lateral surfaces.

Procedure

1. The stabilizing hand holds the metatarsal in position.
2. The manipulating hand glides the proximal phalanx in a medial direction.
3. The use of a padded tongue depressor may assist in directing a more precise manipulation.
4. The use of surgical gloves may allow the clinician to obtain a stronger grip by reducing slippage against the patient's skin.

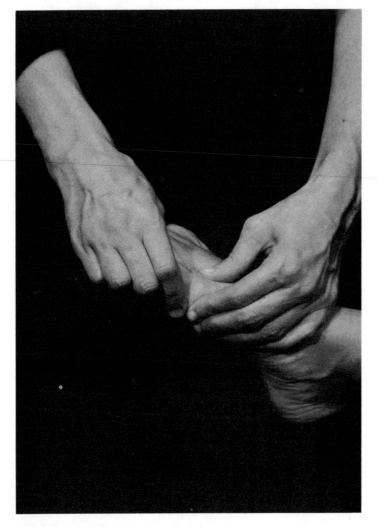

Lateral Glide (Fig 8–28)

Purpose

- To increase joint play in the metatarsophalangeal joints
- To increase range of motion into metatarsophalangeal joint adduction of digits 1 and 2, fibular abduction of digit 3, and abduction of digits 4 and 5
- To decrease pain in the toes
- To increase nutrition to articular structures

Positioning

1. The patient is supine.
2. The metatarsophalangeal joint is positioned in the resting position if conservative techniques are indicated or approximating the restricted range if more aggressive techniques are indicated.
3. The clinician is facing the dorsal surface of the foot.
4. The stabilizing hand grips the head of the metatarsal with the thumb on the dorsal surface of the foot and the index finger on the plantar surface of the foot.

5. The manipulating hand grips the proximal end of the proximal phalanx being manipulated on the medial and lateral surfaces.

Procedure

1. The stabilizing hand holds the metatarsal in position.
2. The manipulating hand glides the base of the proximal phalanx in a lateral direction.
3. The use of a padded tongue depressor may assist the clinician in directing a more precise manipulation.
4. The use of surgical gloves may allow the clinician to obtain a stronger grip by reducing slippage against the patient's skin.

Interphalangeal Joints

Osteokinematic degrees of freedom:	1 motion:
	Flexion/extension
Ligaments:	Medial collateral
	Lateral collateral
Joint orientation:	Proximal phalanx: Distal
	Distal phalanx: Proximal
Type of joint:	Synovial
Articular surface anatomy:	Ovoid
	Proximal phalanx: Convex
	Distal phalanx: Concave
Resting position:	Slight flexion
Close-packed position:	Full extension
Capsular pattern of restriction:	Flexion > extension

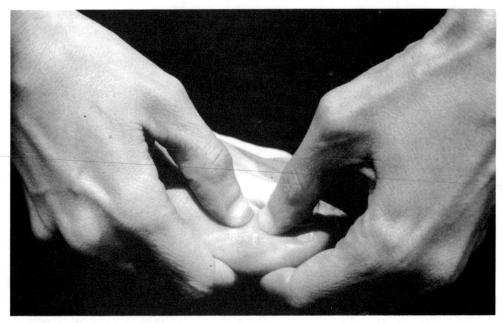

Distraction (Fig 8–29)

Purpose

- To increase joint play in the interphalangeal joints
- To increase overall range of motion in the interphalangeal joints
- To decrease pain in the toes
- To increase nutrition to articular structures

Positioning

1. The patient is supine.
2. The interphalangeal joint is positioned in the resting position if conservative techniques are indicated or approximating the restricted range if more aggressive techniques are indicated.
3. The clinician is facing the dorsal surface of the foot.
4. The stabilizing hand grips the distal end of the proximal phalanx of the joint to be manipulated with the thumb on the dorsal surface of the foot and the index finger on the plantar surface of the foot.
5. The manipulating hand grips the proximal end of the distal phalanx of the joint to be manipulated with the thumb on the dorsal surface of the foot and the index finger on the plantar surface of the foot.

Procedure

1. The stabilizing hand holds the proximal phalanx in position.
2. The manipulating hand moves the distal phalanx distally.
3. The use of a padded tongue depressor may assist the clinician in directing a more precise manipulation.
4. The use of surgical gloves may allow the clinician to obtain a stronger grip by reducing slippage against the patient's skin.

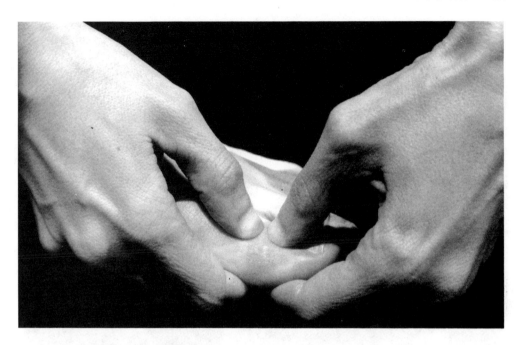

Dorsal Glide (Fig 8–30)

Purpose

- To increase joint play in the interphalangeal joints
- To increase range of motion into interphalangeal extension
- To decrease pain in the toes
- To increase nutrition to articular structures

Positioning

1. The patient is supine.
2. The interphalangeal joint is positioned in the resting position if conservative techniques are indicated or approximating the restricted range if more aggressive techniques are indicated.
3. The clinician is facing the dorsal surface of the foot.
4. The stabilizing hand grips distal end of the proximal phalanx of the joint to be manipulated with the thumb on the dorsal surface of the foot and the index finger on the plantar surface of the foot.
5. The manipulating hand grips the proximal end of the distal phalanx of the joint to be manipulated with the thumb on the dorsal surface of the foot and the index finger on the plantar surface of the foot.

Procedure

1. The stabilizing hand holds the proximal phalanx in position.
2. The manipulating hand glides the distal phalanx in a dorsal direction.
3. The use of a padded tongue depressor may assist the clinician in directing a more precise manipulation.
4. The use of surgical gloves may allow the clinician to obtain a stronger grip by reducing slippage against the patient's skin.

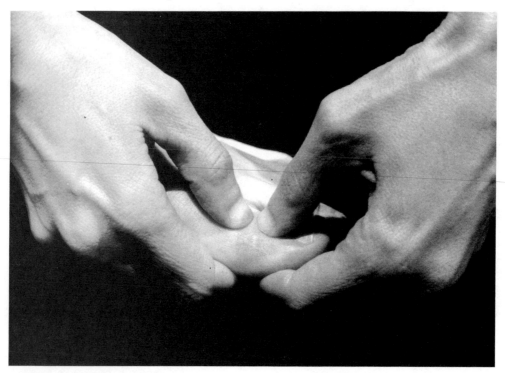

Plantar Glide (Fig 8–31)

Purpose

- To increase joint play in the interphalangeal joints
- To increase range of motion into interphalangeal flexion
- To decrease pain in the toes
- To increase nutrition to articular structures

Positioning

1. The patient is supine.
2. The interphalangeal joint is positioned in the resting position if conservative techniques are indicated or approximating the restricted range if more aggressive techniques are indicated.
3. The clinician is facing the dorsal surface of the foot.
4. The stabilizing hand grips distal end of the proximal phalanx of the joint to be manipulated with the thumb on the dorsal surface of the foot and the index finger on the plantar surface of the foot.
5. The manipulating hand grips the proximal end of the distal phalanx of the joint to be manipulated with the thumb on the dorsal surface of the foot and the index finger on the plantar surface of the foot.

Procedure

1. The stabilizing hand holds the proximal phalanx in position.
2. The manipulating hand glides the distal phalanx in a plantar direction.
3. The use of a padded tongue depressor may assist the clinician in directing a more precise manipulation.

4. The use of surgical gloves may allow the clinician to obtain a stronger grip by reducing slippage against the patient's skin.

REFERENCES

1. Blakeslee TJ, Morris JL: Cuboid syndrome and the significance of midtarsal joint stability. *J Am Podiatr Med Assoc* 1987; 77:638.
2. Brown LP, Yavorsky P: Locomotor biomechanics and pathomechanics: A review. *J Orthop Sports Phys Ther* 1987; 9:3.
3. Donatelli R: Normal biomechanics of the foot and ankle. *J Orthop Sports Phys Ther* 1985; 7:91.
4. Manter JT: Movements of the subtalar and transverse tarsal joints. *Anat Rec* 1941; 80:397.
5. McPoil TG, Knecht HG: Biomechanics of the foot in walking: A functional approach. *J Orthop Sports Phys Ther* 1985; 7:69.
6. Morris JM: Biomechanics of the foot and ankle. *Clin Orthop* 1977; 122:10.
7. Perry J: Anatomy and biomechanics of the hindfoot. *Clin Orthop* 1983; 177:9.
8. Root ML, Orien WP, Weed JH: *Normal and Abnormal Function of the Foot.* Los Angeles, Clinical Biomechanics Corp, 1977.
9. Shereff MJ, Bejjani FJ, Kummer FJ: Kinematics of the first metatarsophalangeal joint. *J Bone Joint Surg [Am]* 1986; 68:392.
10. Soderberg GL: *Kinesiology.* Baltimore, Williams & Wilkins Co, 1986.

Figure **9 – 1**

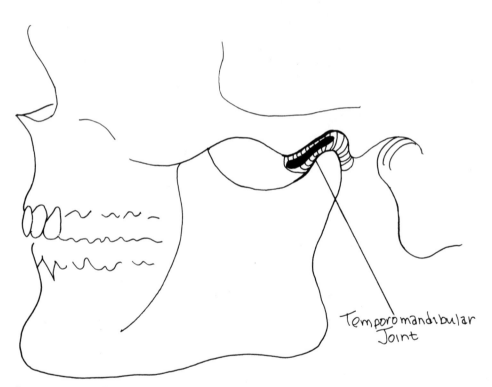

Temporomandibular
Joint

Temporomandibular Joint

Chapter 9

Temporomandibular Joint

Motion in one temporomandibular joint is linked mechanically to motion in the same joint on the opposite side of the body. The joint surface is structurally biconvex, because the convex mandible articulates with the articular eminence of the fossa, which also is convex. The disc is biconcave,[8] and divides the joint into two chambers, creating two concave-convex articulations within the temporomandibular joint.[5] The lower joint, consisting of the mandible caudally and the disc cranially, is primarily responsible for rotation, and the upper joint, consisting of the disc caudally and the temporalis cranially, is primarily responsible for translation.[5, 7] The articular surface anatomy of the upper jaw is of most importance to clinicians treating with joint manipulations, as this is the area where gliding predominates. This joint consists of a convex temporalis on a concave disc; therefore gliding occurs in the same direction as the physiologic motion. As the mandibular condyle moves forward with jaw motion, the disc follows, although disc movement is about half that of the condyle.[2, 6]

Range of motion is considered functional for most jaw activities if 40 mm of opening is present. This should be comprised of approximately 25 mm of rotation and 15 mm of translation.[5] The temporomandibular ligaments are responsible for limiting joint motion in all directions.[1]

OPENING

During jaw opening, rotation and translation occur simultaneously and at a similar ratio to one another throughout range of motion.[4] When evaluating for range of motion into jaw opening, the relative contribution of these two motions should be analyzed. If translation is perceived as deficient, ventral gliding is the primary arthrokinematic motion to be restored. Ventral gliding is somewhat less helpful in restoring the rotational component of opening. Distraction combined with passive range of motion techniques into rotation is more effective in restoring this motion.

PROTRACTION AND RETRACTION

Protraction and retraction occur via a gliding motion, with minimal if any rotation. Ventral gliding manipulation is therefore important in restoring protraction. Retraction rarely is limited.

SIDE GLIDING

With side-gliding, the side to which the motion is occurring rotates and shifts laterally slightly, and the opposite side glides forward, medially, and downward.[3] Side-gliding mobility is restored by performing manipulating glides in which the mandible is moved toward the side opposite the restricted joint.

Temporomandibular Joint

Osteokinematic degrees freedom:	3 motions:
	Opening/closing
	Protraction/retraction
	Side gliding
Ligaments:	Temporomandibular ligament
	Sphenomandibular ligament
	Stylomandibular ligament
Joint orientation:	Temporalis: Caudal, ventral, lateral
	Mandible: Cranial, dorsal, medial
Type of joint:	Synovial
Articular surface anatomy:	Ovoid
	Temporalis: Convex, articulating with a concave disc
	Mandible: Convex, articulating with a concave disc
Resting position:	Mouth slightly opened
Close-packed: Position:	Mouth closed with teeth clenched
Capsular pattern of restriction:	Limitation of mouth opening

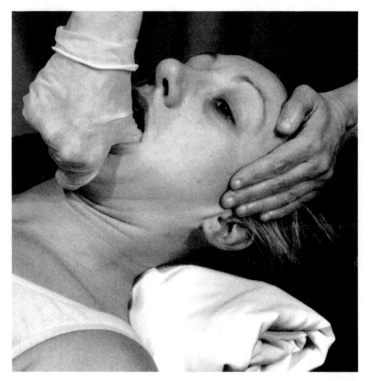

Distraction: First Technique (Fig 9–2)

Purpose

- To increase joint play in the temporomandibular joint
- To increase overall range of motion in the temporomandibular joint
- To decrease pain in the jaw
- To increase nutrition to articular structures

Positioning

1. The patient is supine.
2. The temporomandibular joint is positioned in the resting position if conservative techniques are indicated or approximating the restricted range if more aggressive techniques are indicated.
3. The clinician is standing at the patient's head facing the temporomandibular joint.
4. The clinician should wear surgical gloves to protect both the clinician and patient from transmission of infection.
5. The stabilizing hand supports the head laterally on the same side as the joint being manipulated.
6. The manipulating hand is positioned with the thumb over the lower molars and the fingers wrapped around the lateral lower jaw on the side to be manipulated.

Procedure

1. The stabilizing hand holds the head in position.
2. The manipulating hand moves the mandible caudally with the thumb and guides the movement with the fingers.

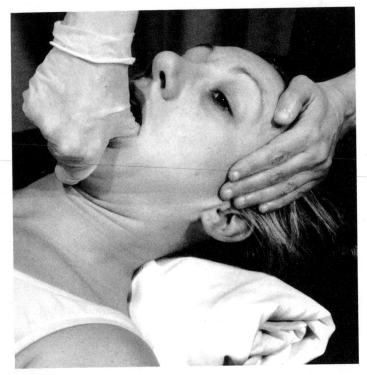

Ventral Glide |(Fig 9-3)

Purpose

- To increase joint play in the temporomandibular joint
- To increase range of motion into translation with temporomandibular opening
- To increase range of motion into temporomandibular protrusion
- To decrease pain in the jaw
- To increase nutrition to articular structures

Positioning

1. The patient is supine.
2. The temporomandibular joint is positioned in the resting position if conservative techniques are indicated or approximating the restricted range if more aggressive techniques are indicated.
3. The clinician is standing at the patient's head facing the temporomandibular joint.
4. The clinician should wear surgical gloves to protect both the clinician and patient from transmission of infection.
5. The stabilizing hand supports the head laterally and ventrally on the same side as the joint being manipulated.
6. The manipulating hand is positioned with the thumb over the lower molars and the fingers wrapped around the lateral lower jaw on the side to be manipulated.

Procedure

1. The stabilizing hand holds the head in position.
2. The manipulating hand glides the mandible in a ventral direction with the thumb and guides the movement with the fingers.

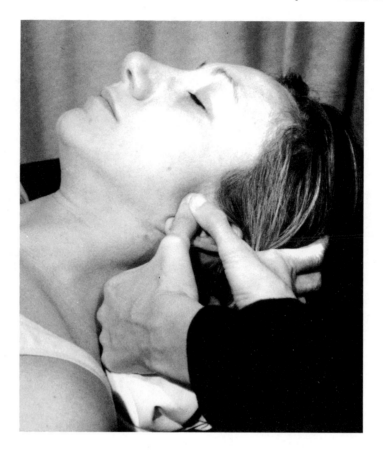

Medial Glide (Fig 9–4)

Purpose

- To increase joint play in the temporomandibular joint
- To increase range of motion into temporomandibular side gliding opposite the side of the manipulating hand
- To decrease pain in the jaw
- To increase nutrition to articular structures

Positioning

1. The patient is supine.
2. The temporomandibular joint is positioned in the resting position if conservative techniques are indicated or approximating the restricted range if more aggressive techniques are indicated.
3. The clinician is standing at the patient's head facing the temporomandibular joint.
4. The manipulating hand is positioned with the thumb over the guiding hand.
5. The guiding hand is positioned with the thumb on the mandibular condyle.

Procedure

1. The manipulating hand glides the mandible in a medial direction with the thumb.
2. The guiding hand controls the position of the manipulating hand.

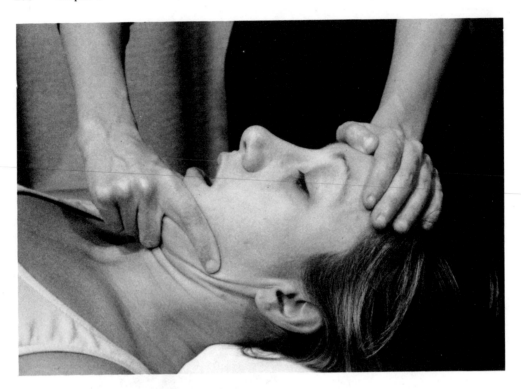

Rocking Mobilization (Fig 9–5)

Purpose

- To increase joint play in the temporomandibular joint
- To increase range of motion into temporomandibular side gliding to the same side as the jaw motion
- To decrease pain in the jaw
- To increase nutrition to articular structures

Positioning

1. The patient is supine.
2. The temporomandibular joint is in the resting position.
3. The clinician is standing at the patient's head facing the temporomandibular joint.
4. The stabilizing hand supports the head laterally on the same side as the jaw motion.
5. The manipulating hand is positioned with the web space over the ventral surface of the chin.

Procedure

1. The stabilizing hand holds the head in position.
2. The manipulating hand glides the mandible laterally away from the side being manipulated.

REFERENCES

1. Burch JG: Activity of the accessory ligaments of the temporomandibular joint. *J Prosthet Dent* 1970; 24:621.
2. Friedman MH, Weisberg J: Application of orthopedic principles in evaluation of the temporomandibular joint. *Phys Ther* 1982; 62:597.
3. Helland MM: Anatomy and function of the temporomandibular joint. *J Orthop Sports Phys Ther* 1980; 1:145.
4. Merlini L, Palla S: The relationship between condylar rotation and anterior translation in healthy and clicking temporomandibular joints. *Schweiz Monatsschr Zahnmed* 1988; 98:1191.
5. Pertes RA et al: The temporomandibular joint in function and dysfunction. *Clin Prev Dent* 1988; 10:23.
6. Rees LA, Lond BSD: The structure and function of the mandibular joint. *Br Dent J* 1954; 46:125.
7. Rocabado M: Arthrokinematics of the temporomandibular joint. *Dent Clin North Am* 1983; 27:573.
8. Scheman P: The condyle fossa relationship: A new look at the anatomy of the human TMJ. *NY State Dent J* 53:25, 1987.

Figure 10–1

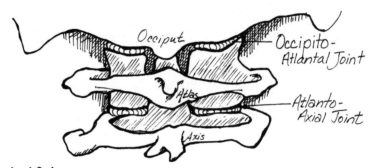

Upper Cervical Spine

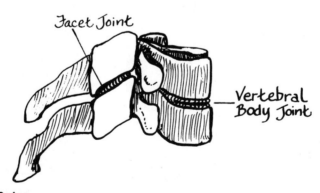

Lower Cervical Spine

Chapter 10

Cervical Spine

The cervical spine is divided into upper and lower components.

FORWARD BENDING AND BACKWARD BENDING

Forward bending and backward bending are the primary motions occurring at the occipitoatlantal joint. This joint accounts for 15 degrees of motion in the sagittal plane.[5] Movement occurs primarily by a rolling motion of the occiput on the atlas.[3] About 10 degrees of forward and backward bending occur at the atlantoaxial joint.[5] Motion into full forward and backward bending is completed by the lower cervical spine. The majority of lower cervical forward and backward bending takes place at the C5-6 interspace. Lower cervical spine motion is guided by the facet joints, which are angulated 45 degrees ventrally from the frontal plane. Because of this angulation, forward bending occurs as the caudal facets of the more cranial vertebra glide up and forward on the cranial facets of the more caudal vertebra.[1] Backward bending is associated with a downward and backward gliding of the more cranial facets on the more caudal facets. The oblique angulation of the facet joints also produces a ventral translation of the more cranial vertebra with forward bending, and conversely, a dorsal translation of the more cranial vertebra with backward bending.

SIDE BENDING AND ROTATION

Approximately 10 degrees of side bending occur at the occipitoatlantal joint, and 5 degrees at the atlantoaxial joint.[5] Rotation is negligible at the occipitoatlantal joint, but the atlantoaxial joint is capable of a full 50 degrees of rotation in each direction.[5] Rotation at the atlantoaxial joint is thought to be coupled with side bending at the occipitoatlantal joint to the same side, although the research regarding this is not conclusive.[3, 6] Atlantoaxial rotation is accompanied by a vertical translation of the atlas in a caudal direction at the end of rotation.[4, 5, 7]

Rotation at the atlantoaxial joint can restrict blood flow in the vertebral arteries. It therefore is crucial that the clinician test for signs of potential vertebral artery occlusion before proceeding with any of the techniques described for the upper cervical spine or any of the lower cervical spine techniques involving neck movement.

Most of the motion for side bending occurs at the lower cervical spine.[1] Excessive side bending is blocked by the uncovertebral joints. The lower cervical spine also is responsible for approximately 45 degrees of rotation in either direction. Most of the movement for lower cervical side bending and rotation occur at the C5-6 interspace. As with forward bending, lower cervical side bending and rotation are guided by the angulation of the facet joints. This angulation produces a strong coupling motion consisting of side bending and rotation to the same side.[2, 7] The more cranial articulation on the side to which side bending and rotation are occurring glides down and back as the contralateral articulation glides up and forward. Side bending and rotation at the lower cervical spine thus are incapable of occurring independent of one another. When a person side bends or rotates at the neck, he or she actually is side bending and rotating at the lower cervical spine and compensating for the coupled motion by movement at the upper cervical spine.[1] Limitations in side bending are accompanied by limitations in rotation to the same side. When the clinician performs a technique to increase joint play into either rotation or side bending, that technique also produces an increase in the coupled motion.

Upper Cervical Spine (Occiput Through C2)

Osteokinematic degrees of freedom:	Occipitoatlantal joint: 3 motions:
	Forward/backward bending
	Side bending
	Rotation
	Atlantoaxial joint: 3 motions:
	Rotation
	Forward/backward bending
	Side bending
Ligaments:	Tectorial membrane
	Ligamentum nuchae
	Alar ligament
	Transverse ligament
	Apical ligament
	Interspinous ligament
	Supraspinous ligament
	Anterior longitudinal ligament
	Posterior longitudinal ligament
Joint orientation:	Occiput: Caudal
	Atlas cranial surface: Cranial
	Atlas caudal facet: Caudal, medial
	Axis cranial facet: Cranial, lateral
	Atlas also encircles the odontoid process of the axis
Type of joint:	Synovial
Articular surface anatomy:	Ovoid
	Occiput: Convex
	Atlas cranial surface: Concave
	Atlas caudal facet: Convex
	Axis cranial facet: Convex
	Atlas and axis also articulate via the odontoid process
Resting position:	Not described
Close-packed Position:	Not described
Capsular pattern of restriction:	Occipitoatlantal joint: Forward bending > backward bending
	Atlantoaxial joint: Restriction with rotation

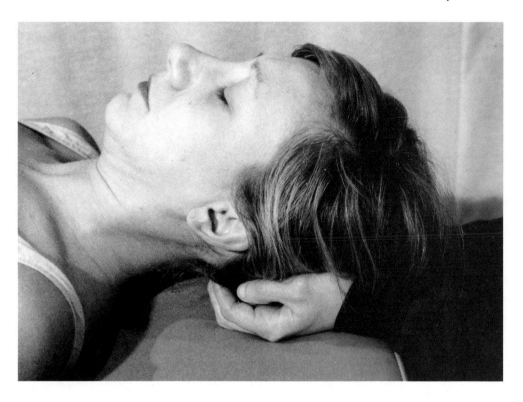

Distraction (Fig 10–2)

Purpose

- To increase joint play in the upper cervical spine
- To increase overall range of motion in the upper cervical spine
- To decrease pain in the upper neck region
- To increase nutrition to articular structures

Positioning

1. The patient is supine.
2. The joint is positioned midway between forward bending and backward bending.
3. The clinician is sitting at the patient's head facing the patient.
4. Vertebral artery testing should be done before performing this or any other manipulation techniques on the upper cervical spine.
5. Both hands are positioned with the fingertips immediately caudal to the base of the occiput and the hands on the dorsal surface of the skull

Procedure

1. Both fingers glide the occiput cranially, thus lifting the skull away from the clinician's palms and allowing the weight of the head to distract the occiput from the cervical spine.
2. This position can be maintained for several minutes to maximally stretch suboccipital tissue.
3. This technique also effectively stretches the suboccipital musculature.

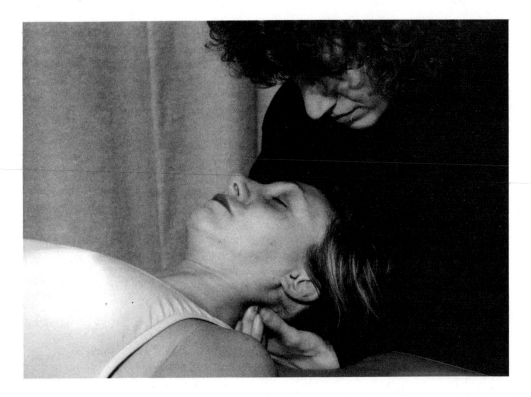

Forward Bending Manipulation (Fig 10–3)

Purpose

- To increase joint play in the upper cervical spine
- To increase range of motion into forward bending at the upper cervical spine
- To decrease pain in the upper neck region
- To increase nutrition to articular structures

Positioning

1. The patient is supine.
2. The joint is positioned midway between forward bending and backward bending.
3. The clinician is sitting at the patient's head facing the patient.
4. Vertebral artery testing should be done before performing this or any other manipulation techniques on the upper cervical spine.
5. The stabilizing hand grips the axis dorsally with the web space and laterally with the fingers.
6. The manipulating hand grips the occiput dorsally with the web space.

Procedure

1. The stabilizing hand holds the axis in position.
2. The manipulating hand glides the occiput cranially, thus allowing the head to move into forward bending.

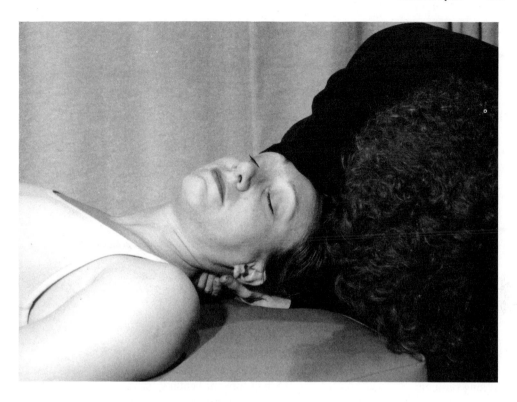

Rotation Manipulation (Fig 10–4)

Purpose

- To increase joint play in the upper cervical spine
- To increase range of motion into rotation at the upper cervical spine to the same side as the side to which the head is turned
- To decrease pain in the upper neck region
- To increase nutrition to articular structures

Positioning

1. The patient is supine.
2. The joint is positioned in slight rotation.
3. The clinician is at the patient's head facing the patient with the clinician's shoulder positioned on the patient's forehead.
4. Vertebral artery testing should be done before performing this or any other manipulation techniques on the upper cervical spine.
5. The stabilizing hand grips the axis dorsally with the web space and laterally with the fingers.
6. The manipulating hand grips the occiput dorsally.

Procedure

1. The stabilizing hand holds the axis in position.
2. The manipulating hand glides the occiput into rotation as the shoulder guides the motion.

Lower Cervical Spine (C3 Through T2)

Osteokinematic degrees of freedom:	Three motions: 　Forward/backward bending 　Side bending 　Rotation
Ligaments:	Anterior longitudinal ligament Posterior longitudinal ligament Supraspinous ligament Interspinous ligament Ligamentum flavum Intertransverse ligament
Joint orientation:	Caudal facet of cranial vertebra: Caudal, 　ventral, lateral Cranial facet of caudal vertebra: Cranial, 　dorsal, medial Cranial vertebral body: Caudal Caudal vertebral body: Cranial
Type of joint:	Facets: Synovial Disc: Amphiarthrodial
Articular surface anatomy:	Ovoid, plane Cranial facet: Convex Caudal facet: Concave
Resting position:	Slight forward bending
Close-packed position:	Full backward bending
Capsular pattern of restriction:	Side bending = rotation > back bending

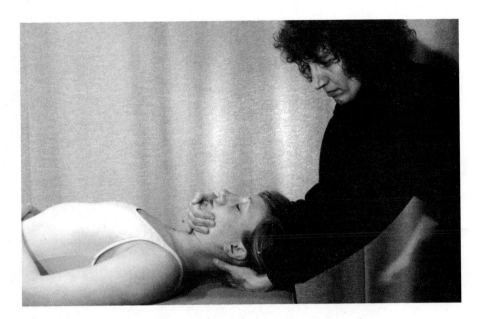

Distraction (Fig 10–5)

Purpose

- To increase joint play in the cervical spine
- To increase overall of motion in the cervical spine
- To decrease pain in the lower neck region
- To increase nutrition to articular structures

Positioning

1. The patient is supine.
2. The joint is in the resting position.
3. The clinician is standing at the patient's head facing the patient.
4. The manipulating hand grips the occiput dorsally with the web space.
5. The guiding hand gently grips the chin.

Procedure

1. The clinician leans backward, thus moving the cervical spine in a cranial direction.
2. Most of the force exerted by the clinician should be directed to the occiput because excessive pressure on the chin may cause the patient to develop temporomandibular joint problems.

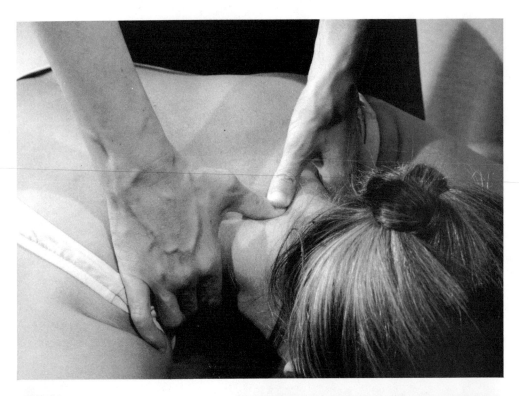

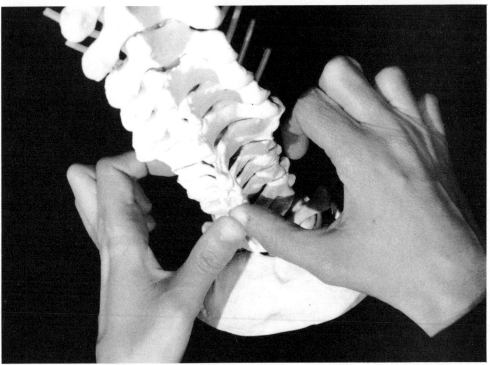

Ventral Glide (Figs 10–6, 10–7)

Purpose

- To increase joint play in the lower cervical spine
- To increase overall range of motion in the lower cervical spine
- To decrease pain in the lower cervical region
- To increase nutrition to articular structures

Positioning

1. The patient is supine or prone.
2. The cervical spine is in the resting position if conservative techniques are indicated or approximating the restricted range if more aggressive techniques are indicated.
3. The clinician is at the patient's head facing the cervical spine.
4. The manipulating hand is positioned with the thumb over the thumb of the guiding hand.
5. The guiding hand is positioned with the thumb over the spinous process being manipulated.

Procedure

1. The manipulating hand glides the spinous process ventrally.
2. The guiding hand controls the position of the manipulating hand.

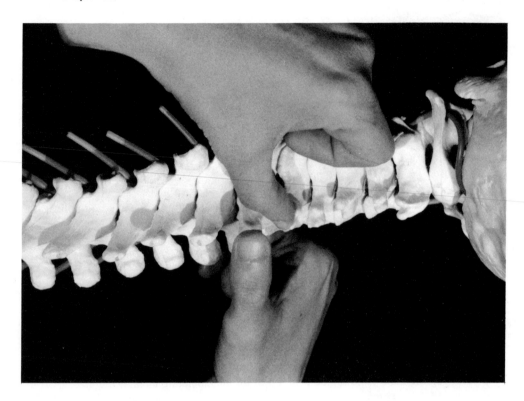

Cranial Glide: First Technique (Fig 10–8)

Purpose

- To increase joint play in the lower cervical spine
- To increase range of motion into forward bending at the lower cervical spine
- To reduce a backward bent positional fault in the lower cervical spine
- To decrease pain in the lower cervical region
- To increase nutrition to articular structures

Positioning

1. The patient is supine or prone.
2. The cervical spine is in the resting position if conservative techniques are indicated or approximating the restricted range if more aggressive techniques are indicated.
3. The clinician is at the patient's head facing the cervical spine.
4. The stabilizing hand is positioned with the thumb on the spinous process of the more caudal vertebra.
5. The manipulating hand is positioned with the thumb over the most caudal surface of the spinous process of the more cranial vertebra.

Procedure

1. The stabilizing hand holds the vertebra in position.
2. The manipulating hand glides the spinous process cranially and ventrally.

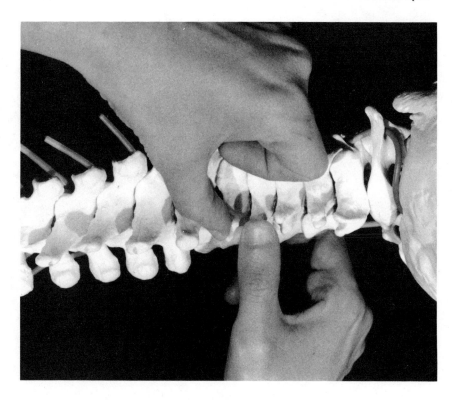

Cranial Glide: Second Technique (Fig 10–9)

Purpose

- To increase joint play in the lower cervical spine
- To increase range of motion into backward bending in the lower cervical spine
- To reduce a forward bent positional fault in the lower cervical spine
- To decrease pain in the lower cervical region
- To increase nutrition to articular structures

Positioning

1. The patient is supine or prone.
2. The cervical spine is in the resting position if conservative techniques are indicated or approximating the restricted range if more aggressive techniques are indicated.
3. The clinician is at the patient's head facing the cervical spine.
4. The stabilizing hand is positioned with the thumb on the spinous process of the more cranial vertebra
5. The manipulating hand is positioned with the thumb over the most caudal surface of the spinous process of the more caudal vertebra.

Procedure

1. The stabilizing hand holds the vertebra in position.
2. The manipulating hand glides the spinous process cranially and ventrally.

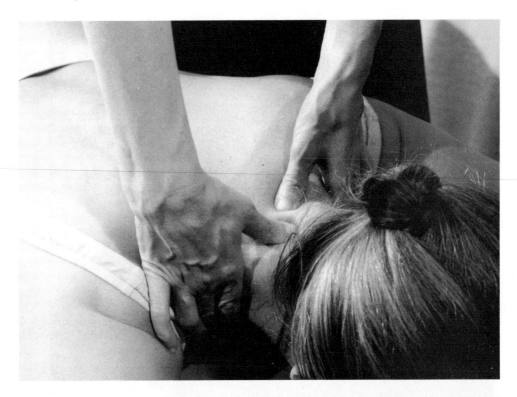

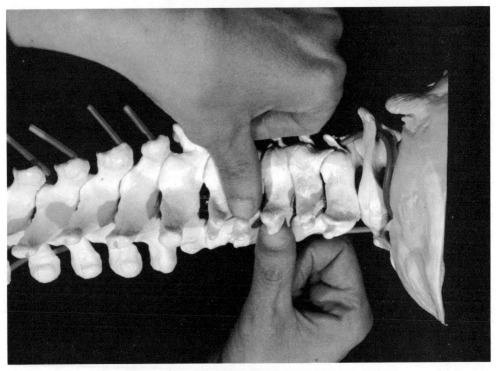

Rotation Manipulation: First Technique (Figs 10–10, 10–11)

Purpose

- To increase joint play in the lower cervical spine
- To increase range of motion into lower cervical rotation and side bending to the same side as the side of the manipulating hand
- To reduce a cervical rotational or side bent positional fault, which is positioned toward the direction opposite the side of the manipulating hand
- To decrease pain in the lower cervical region
- To increase nutrition to articular structures

Positioning

1. The patient is supine or prone.
2. The cervical spine is in the resting position if conservative techniques are indicated or approximating the restricted range if more aggressive techniques are indicated.
3. The clinician is at the patient's head facing the cervical spine.
4. The stabilizing hand is positioned with the thumb on the lateral surface of the spinous process of the more caudal vertebra opposite the side to which the vertebra is being manipulated.
5. The manipulating hand is positioned with the thumb on the lateral surface of the spinous process of the more cranial vertebra on the same side as the side to which the vertebra is being manipulated.

Procedure

1. The stabilizing hand holds the more caudal vertebra in position.
2. The manipulating hand glides the more cranial spinous process in a medial direction, thus rotating and side bending the vertebra being manipulated on the vertebra below it.

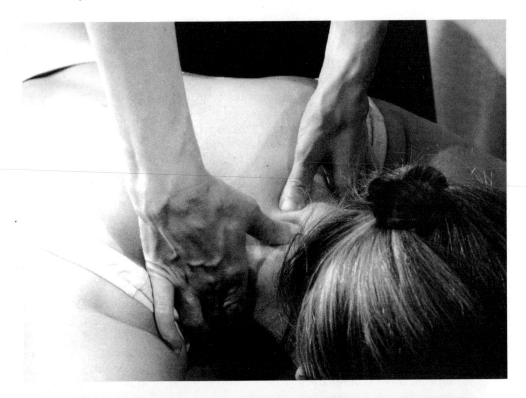

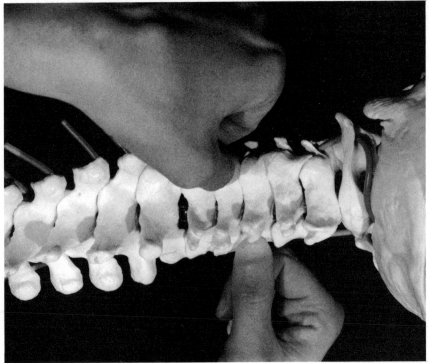

Rotation Manipulation: Second Technique (Figs 10–12, 10–13)

Purpose

- To increase joint play in the lower cervical spine
- To increase range of motion into lower cervical rotation and side bending opposite the side of the manipulating hand
- To reduce a cervical rotational or side bent positional fault, which is positioned toward the same side as the side of the manipulating hand
- To decrease pain in the lower cervical region
- To increase nutrition to articular structures

Positioning

1. The patient is supine or prone.
2. The cervical spine is in the resting position if conservative techniques are indicated or approximating the restricted range if more aggressive techniques are indicated.
3. The clinician is at the patient's head facing the cervical spine.
4. The stabilizing hand is positioned with the thumb on the facet joint of the more caudal vertebra on the same side as the side to which the vertebra is being manipulated.
5. The manipulating hand is positioned with the thumb on the facet joint of the more cranial vertebra opposite the side to which the vertebra is being manipulated.

Procedure

1. The stabilizing hand holds the more caudal vertebra in position.
2. The manipulating hand glides the more cranial facet joint in a ventral and cranial direction, thus rotating and side bending the vertebra being manipulated on the vertebra below it.

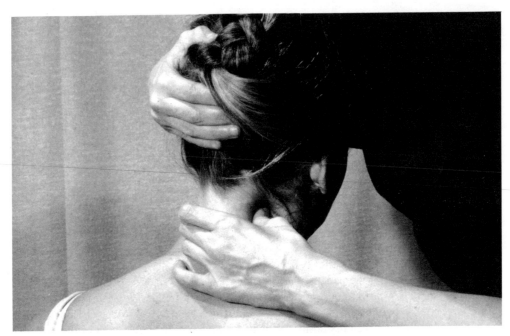

Rotation Manipulation: Third Technique (Fig 10–14)

Purpose

- To increase joint play in the lower cervical spine
- To increase range of motion into lower cervical rotation and side bending to the same side as the side to which the head is turned
- To reduce a cervical rotational or side bent positional fault, which is positioned toward the direction opposite the side to which the head is turned
- To release impinged meniscoid tissue
- To decrease pain in the lower cervical region
- To increase nutrition to articular structures

Positioning

1. The patient is sitting.
2. The cervical spine is in the resting position.
3. The clinician is at the patient's side facing the patient with the clinician's arm supporting the patient's head.
4. The clinician locks the more cranial vertebra by forward bending the neck or side bending and/or rotating the neck to the same side as the direction of the manipulation to the extent that the motion segment above the one being manipulated is fully forward bent, side bent, and/or rotated, but the motion segment being manipulated has not yet moved.
5. The stabilizing hand grips the more caudal vertebra dorsally with the web space and laterally with the fingers.

Procedure

1. The stabilizing hand holds the caudal vertebra in position.
2. The manipulating hand rotates the patient's head.

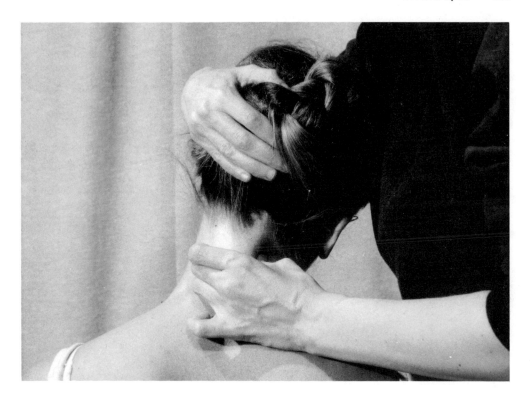

Side Bending Manipulation (Fig 10–15)

Purpose

- To increase joint play in the lower cervical spine
- To increase range of motion into lower cervical side bending and rotation to the same side as the side to which the head is bent
- To reduce a cervical side bent or rotational positional fault, which is positioned toward the direction opposite the side to which the head is bent
- To decrease pain in the lower cervical region
- To increase nutrition to articular structures

Positioning

1. The patient is sitting.
2. The cervical spine is in the resting position.
3. The clinician is at the patient's side facing the patient with the clinician's arm supporting the patient's head.
4. The clinician locks the more cranial vertebra by forward bending the neck or side bending and/or rotating the neck to the same side as the direction of the manipulation to the extent that the motion segment above the one being manipulated is fully forward bent, side bent, and/or rotated, but the motion segment being manipulated has not yet moved.
5. The stabilizing hand grips the more caudal vertebra dorsally with the web space and laterally with the fingers.

Procedure

1. The stabilizing hand holds the caudal vertebra in position.
2. The manipulating hand side bends the patient's head.

REFERENCES

1. Fielding JW: Normal and selected abnormal motion of the cervical spine from the second cervical vertebra to the seventh cervical vertebra based on cineroentgenography. *J Bone Joint Surg* 1964; 46-A:1779.
2. Goel VK et al: An in-vitro study of the kinematics of the normal, injured and stabilized cervical spine. *J Biomechanics* 1984; 17:363.
3. Grieve GP: *Common Vertebral Joint Problems,* ed 2. New York, Churchill Livingstone, 1988.
4. Hohl M: Normal motions in the upper portion of the cervical spine. *J Bone Joint Surg* 1964; 46A:1777.
5. Magee D: Orthopedic physical assessment. Philadelphia, WB Saunders, 1987.
6. Soderberg GL: *Kinesiology.* Baltimore, Williams & Wilkins, 1986.
7. White AA, Panjabi MM: *Clinical Biomechanics of the Spine,* ed 2. Philadelphia, JB Lippincott Co, 1990.

Figure **11–1**

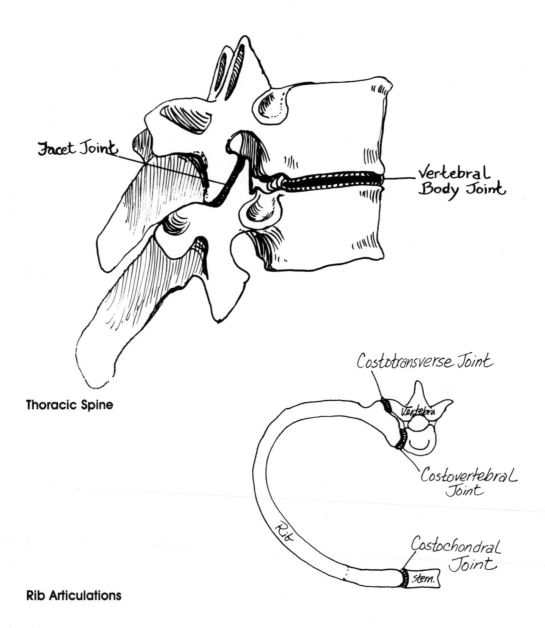

Facet Joint

Vertebral
Body Joint

Thoracic Spine

Costotransverse Joint

Vertebra

Costovertebral
Joint

Rib

Costochondral
Joint

stern.

Rib Articulations

Chapter 11

Thoracic Spine and Ribs

The primary function of the thoracic spine is to provide support to the trunk in the upright position and to protect the spinal cord and vital organs. Despite its role as a stabilizing force, the thoracic spine contributes to 25% of the total movement in the spine. Motion is restricted primarily by the ribs.

FORWARD AND BACKWARD BENDING

The facet joints in the thoracic spine are oriented similarly to those of the cervical spine, with the major exception that they are angulated more cranially and less ventrally. Forward and backward bending are accompanied by a gliding motion between the two facet articulations, similar to that in the cervical spine except that ventral translation is minimal. The amount of forward and backward bending increases in the more caudal segments in relation to the amount of motion in the more cranial segments.[4]

The spinous processes in the thoracic spine are positioned caudally in relation to the motion segment. They therefore can be used as a lever to rotate the vertebral body, resulting in a gliding of the facet articulations that is associated with forward and backward bending in the thoracic spine.

ROTATION AND SIDE BENDING

The relative amount of rotation in the thoracic spine decreases at the more caudal vertebrae. Side bending, on the other hand, increases at the more caudal vertebrae.[4] Coupled motion most likely exists in the thoracic spine, although the extent to which it occurs is much less than in the cervical facets. There is a great deal of inconsistency in the literature regarding the nature of thoracic coupled motion. Motion in the upper thoracic spine most likely mimics that of the cervical spine; thus side bending and rotation are coupled to the same side.[1, 3, 4] Motion in the midthoracic spine is both inconsistent and variable among individuals.[1, 4] The lower thoracic spine most likely begins to resemble the upper lumbar spine in regard to its coupling pattern and therefore is characterized by side bending coupled with rotation to the opposite side.[1] Many clinicians also believe that the patterns of coupled motion are altered with changes in the sagittal plane positioning of the spine. Some research has given credence to this theory by concluding that the angulation of the vertebral bodies determines the coupling pattern in the spine.[3] In segments where the nature of the coupled motion can be identified, limitations in one motion will occur in conjunction with limitations in the coupled motion. Restoring motion in one direction therefore will have some effect on the restoration of motion in the coupled direction. Some clinicians also believe that if a pattern of restriction exists that is consistent with a known coupling pattern that changes with position, the pattern of restriction will be consistent with the position the patient was in when the injury occurred.

Vertebral rotation in the thoracic spine produces an associated movement of the corresponding ribs, due to the rib's attachment to the vertebral bodies and transverse processes. The rib on the side to which the vertebra is rotated moves in a dorsal direction, and the rib opposite the side to which the vertebra is rotated moves in a ventral direction. If a positional fault of the thoracic spine is detected, an associated positional fault of the ribs therefore also should be investigated. Restrictions in rib mobility are also fairly common. Both ventral restrictions and dorsal positional faults can be corrected easily with joint manipulation techniques.

INSPIRATION AND EXPIRATION

Ribs 2 through 5 move primarily in a forward and upward direction with inspiration and in a backward and downward direction with expiration; this is called pump-handle motion. Ribs 7 through 10 move primarily laterally and upward with inspiration and medially and downward with expiration; this is described as bucket-handle motion. Ribs 5 through 7 are transitional ribs and exhibit characteristics of both movements. All of these motions are accompanied by rotation of the ribs around their longitudinal axes.[1] Ribs 11 and 12 are capable of movement but are generally held in a relative position of expiration by the quadratus lumborum muscle. They are capable of lateral movement with inspiration and medial movement with expiration; this is called caliper motion. The first rib moves only minimally, because it is fused to the sternum. A small amount of spinal movement occurs with respiration, but for the most part a large degree of independence exists between motion at the spine and ribs.[2]

Thoracic Spine

Osteokinematic degrees of freedom:	3 motions:
	Forward/backward bending
	Side bending
	Rotation
Ligaments:	Anterior longitudinal ligament
	Posterior longitudinal ligament
	Supraspinous ligament
	Interspinous ligament
	Ligamentum flavum
	Intertransverse ligament
Joint orientation:	Caudal facet of cranial vertebra: Ventral, caudal, medial
	Cranial facet of caudal vertebra: Dorsal, cranial, lateral
	Cranial vertebral body: Caudal
	Caudal vertebral body: Cranial
Type of joint:	Facets: Synovial
	Disc: Amphiarthrodial

Articular surface anatomy: Ovoid, plane
                                     Cranial facet: Convex
                                     Caudal facet: Concave
Resting position: Not described
Close-packed position: Full backward bending
Capsular pattern of restriction: Side bending = rotation > back bending

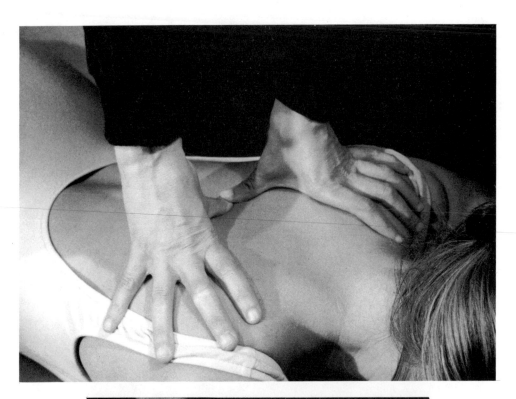

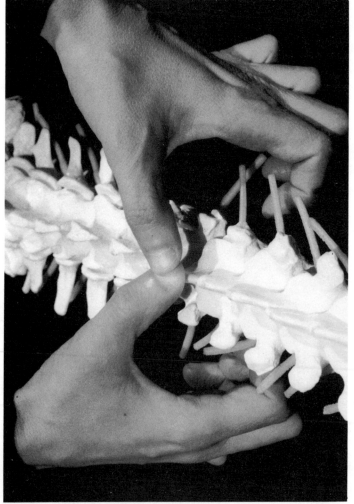

Ventral Glide: First Technique (Figs 11–2, 11–3)

(It is preferable to perform this technique using the heel of the hand as the mobilizing force. The thumb was used to better visualize the joint.)

Purpose

- To increase joint play in the thoracic spine
- To increase range of motion into backward bending between the vertebra being manipulated and the one immediately below and into forward bending between the vertebra being manipulated and the one immediately above
- To reduce a thoracic forward bent positional fault between the vertebra being manipulated and the one immediately below and a thoracic backward bent positional fault between the vertebra being manipulated and the one immediately above
- To decrease pain in the thoracic region
- To increase nutrition to articular structures

Positioning

1. The patient is prone.
2. The thoracic spine is in the resting position.
3. The clinician is standing at the patient's side facing the thoracic spine.
4. The manipulating hand is positioned with the heel of the hand or the thumb over the thumb of the guiding hand.
5. The guiding hand is positioned with the thumb over the spinous process being manipulated.

Procedure

1. The manipulating hand glides the spinous process ventrally, thus rotating the vertebra into backward bending on the vertebra below and into forward bending on the vertebra above.
2. The guiding hand controls the position of the manipulating hand.

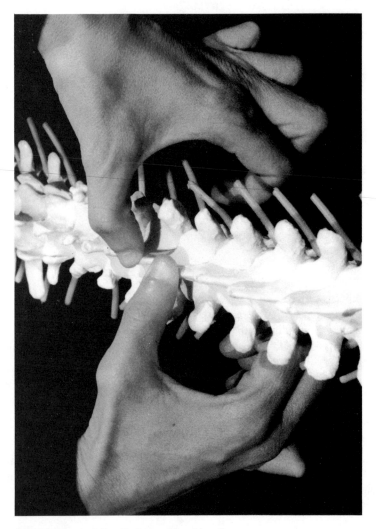

Ventral Glide: Second Technique (Fig 11–4)

(It is preferable to perform this technique using the pisiform as the mobilizing force. The thumb is used to better visualize the joint.)

Purpose

- To increase joint play in the thoracic spine
- To increase range of motion into backward bending between the vertebra being manipulated and the one immediately below
- To reduce a thoracic forward bent positional fault between the vertebra being manipulated and the one immediately below
- To decrease pain in the thoracic region
- To increase nutrition to articular structures

Positioning

1. The patient is prone.
2. The thoracic spine is in the resting position.
3. The clinician is standing at the patient's side facing the thoracic spine.

4. The stabilizing hand is positioned with the thumb on the spinous process of the more caudal vertebra.
5. The manipulating hand is positioned with the pisiform or thumb over the spinous process of the more cranial vertebra.

Procedure

1. The stabilizing hand holds the vertebra in position.
2. The manipulating hand glides the spinous process ventrally, thus rotating the vertebra into backward bending on the vertebra below.

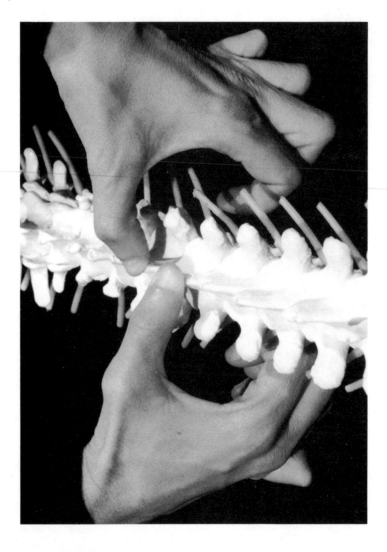

Ventral Glide: Third Technique (Fig 11−5)

(It is preferable to perform this technique using the pisiform as the immobilizing force. The thumb was used to better visualize the joint.)

Purpose

- To increase joint play in the thoracic spine
- To increase range of motion into forward bending between the vertebra being manipulated and the one immediately above
- To reduce a thoracic backward bent positional fault between the vertebra being manipulated and the one immediately above
- To decrease pain in the thoracic region
- To increase nutrition to articular structures

Positioning

1. The patient is prone.
2. The thoracic spine is in the resting position.

3. The clinician is standing at the patient's side facing the thoracic spine.
4. The stabilizing hand is positioned with the thumb on the spinous process of the more cranial vertebra.
5. The manipulating hand is positioned with the pisiform or thumb over the spinous process of the more caudal vertebra.

Procedure

1. The stabilizing hand holds the vertebra in position.
2. The manipulating hand glides the spinous process ventrally, thus rotating the vertebra into forward bending on the vertebra above.

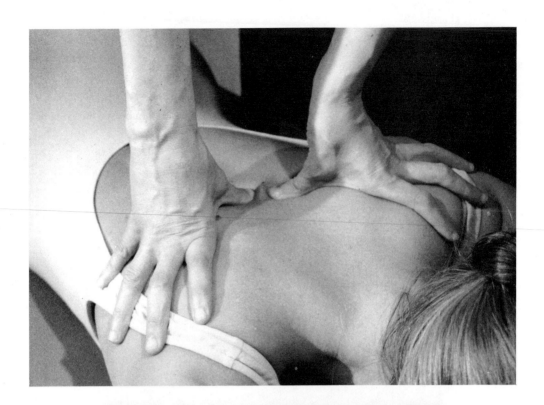

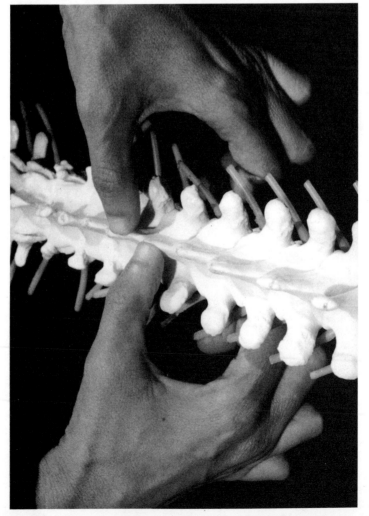

Rotation Manipulation: First Technique (Figs 11–6, 11–7)

Purpose

- To increase joint play in the thoracic spine
- To increase range of motion into thoracic rotation to the same side as the side of the manipulating hand
- To reduce a thoracic rotational positional fault, which is positioned toward the direction opposite the side of the manipulating hand
- To decrease pain in the thoracic region
- To increase nutrition to articular structures

Positioning

1. The patient is prone.
2. The thoracic spine is in the resting position.
3. The clinician is standing at the patient's side facing the thoracic spine.
4. The stabilizing hand is positioned with the thumb on the lateral surface of the spinous process of the more caudal vertebra opposite the side to which the vertebra is being manipulated.
5. The manipulating hand is positioned with the thumb on the lateral surface of the spinous process of the more cranial vertebra on the same side as the side to which the vertebra is being manipulated.

Procedure

1. The stabilizing hand holds the more caudal vertebra in position.
2. The manipulating hand glides the more cranial spinous process in a medial direction, thus rotating the vertebra being manipulated on the vertebra below it.

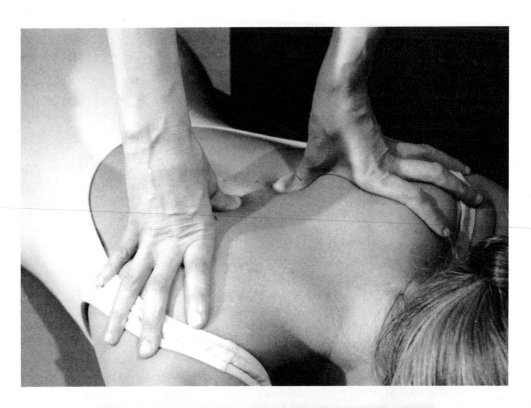

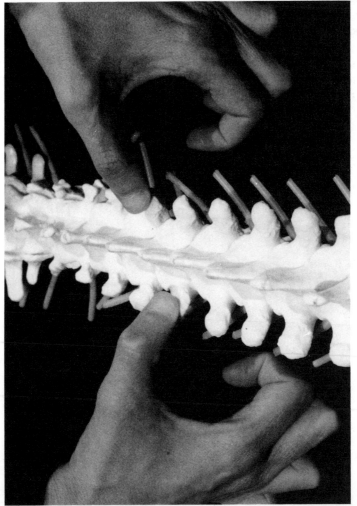

Rotation Manipulation: Second Technique (Figs 11–8, 11–9)

(It is preferable to perform this technique using the pisiform. The thumb was used to better visualize the joint.)

Purpose

- To increase joint play in the thoracic spine
- To increase range of motion into thoracic rotation to the opposite side as the side of the manipulating hand
- To reduce a thoracic rotational positional fault, which is positioned toward the same side as the side of the manipulating hand
- To decrease pain in the thoracic region
- To increase nutrition to articular structures

Positioning

1. The patient is prone.
2. The thoracic spine is in the resting position.
3. The clinician is standing at the patient's side facing the thoracic spine.
4. The stabilizing hand is positioned with the pisiform or thumb on the transverse process of the more caudal vertebra on the same side as the side to which the vertebra is being manipulated.
5. The manipulating hand is positioned with the pisiform or thumb on the transverse process of the more cranial vertebra opposite the side to which the vertebra is being manipulated.

Procedure

1. The stabilizing hand holds the more caudal vertebra in position.
2. The manipulating hand glides the more cranial transverse process in a ventral direction, thus rotating the vertebra being manipulated on the vertebra below it.

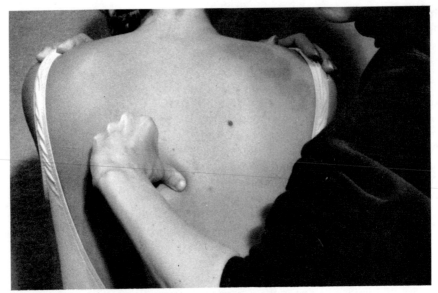

Rotation Manipulation: Third Technique (Fig 11–10)

Purpose

- To increase joint play in the thoracic spine
- To increase range of motion into thoracic rotation to the same side as the side to which the body is turned
- To reduce a thoracic rotational positional fault, which is positioned toward the direction opposite the side to which the trunk is turned
- To release impinged meniscoid tissue
- To decrease pain in the thoracic region
- To increase nutrition to articular structures

Positioning

1. The patient is sitting with his arms positioned across his chest.
2. The thoracic spine is in the resting position.
3. The clinician is at the patient's side facing the patient with the clinician's arm across the patient's chest and the clinician's shoulder and hand supporting the patient's shoulders.
4. The clinician locks the most cranial vertebra by rotating or side bending the upper trunk to the same side as the direction of the manipulation to the extent that the motion segment above the one being manipulated is fully rotated, but the motion segment being manipulated has not yet moved.
5. The stabilizing hand is positioned with the thumb on the lateral surface of the more caudal spinous process on the opposite side of the direction of the manipulation.
6. The manipulating hand is positioned on the shoulder opposite the side of the direction of the manipulation.

Procedure

1. The stabilizing hand holds the caudal vertebra in position.
2. The manipulating hand rotates the patient's trunk.

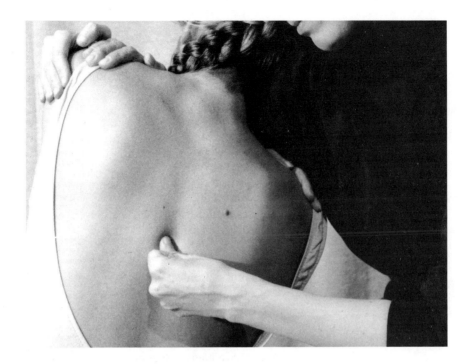

Side Bending Manipulation (Fig 11−11)

Purpose

- To increase joint play in the thoracic spine
- To increase range of motion into thoracic side bending to the same side as the side to which the body is bent
- To reduce a thoracic side bent positional fault, which is positioned toward the direction opposite the side to which the trunk is bent
- To decrease pain in the thoracic region
- To increase nutrition to articular structures

Positioning

1. The patient is sitting with his arms positioned across his chest.
2. The thoracic spine is in the resting position.
3. The clinician is at the patient's side facing the patient with the clinician's arm across the patient's chest and the clinician's shoulder and hand supporting the patient's shoulders.
4. The clinician locks the most cranial vertebra by side bending or rotating the upper trunk to the same side as the direction of the manipulation to the extent that the motion segment above the one being manipulated is fully side bent, but the motion segment being manipulated has not yet moved.
5. The stabilizing hand is positioned with the thumb on the lateral surface of the more caudal spinous process on either side.
6. The manipulating hand is positioned on the shoulder opposite the side of the direction of the manipulation.

Procedure

1. The stabilizing hand holds the caudal vertebra in position.
2. The manipulating hand side bends the patient's trunk.

Rib Articulations

Osteokinematic degrees of freedom:
  3 motions:
  Ventral/dorsal
  Lateral/medial
  Rotation

Ligaments:
  Costovertebral joints:
    Capsular ligament
    Radiate ligament
    Intra-articular ligament
  Costotransverse joints:
    Capsular ligament
    Costotransverse ligament

Joint orientation:
  Vertebral bodies: Dorsal, lateral
  Rib at costovertebral joint: Ventral, medial
  Transverse process: Ventral, lateral
  Rib at costotransverse joint: Dorsal, medial
  Sternum: Lateral, caudal
  Rib at costochondral joint: Medial, cranial

Type of joint:
  Costovertebral joint: Synovial
  Costotransverse joint: Synovial
  Costochondral joint: Synchondrosis

Articular surface anatomy:
  Vertebral bodies: Concave
  Rib at costovertebral joint: Convex
  Transverse process: Concave
  Rib at costotransverse joint: Convex
  Sternum: Concave
  Rib at costochondral joint: Convex

Resting position:
  Not described
Close-packed position:
  Not described
Capsular pattern of restriction:
  Not described

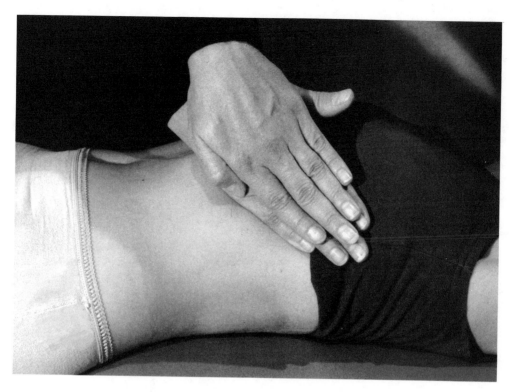

Expiration Manipulation: First Technique (Fig 11–12)

Purpose

- To increase joint play in the articulations at ribs 5 through 7
- To increase range of motion into pump-handle and bucket-handle expiration at ribs 5 through 7
- To reduce an inspiration positional fault in ribs 5 through 7
- To decrease pain in the thoracic area
- To increase nutrition to articular structures

Positioning

1. The patient is supine.
2. The trunk is in midrange position.
3. The clinician is at the patient's side facing the patient's trunk.
4. The manipulating hand is positioned on the anterolateral surface of the trunk with the ulnar border of the hand between the rib being manipulated and the one above.
5. The guiding hand is positioned over the manipulating hand.

Procedure

1. The manipulating hand guides the rib into expiration as the patient exhales and resists inspiration as the patient inhales.
2. The guiding hand controls the position of the manipulating hand.

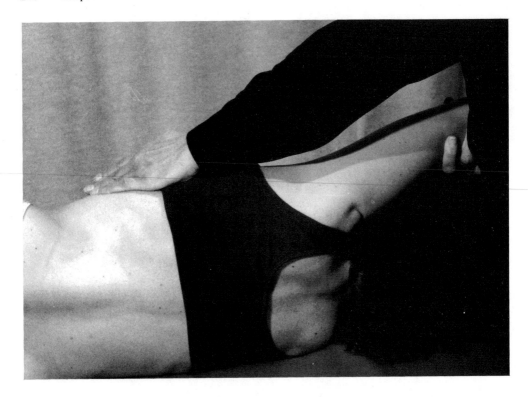

Expiration Manipulation: Second Technique (Fig 11–13)

Purpose

- To increase joint play in the articulations at ribs 7 through 12
- To increase range of motion into bucket-handle expiration at ribs 7 through 12
- To reduce an inspiration positional fault in ribs 7 through 12
- To decrease pain in the thoracic area
- To increase nutrition to articular structures

Positioning

1. The patient is side-lying with the arm positioned over the head.
2. The trunk is in midrange position.
3. The clinician is at the patient's head facing the patient's trunk.
4. The manipulating hand is positioned on the lateral surface of the trunk with the ulnar border of the hand between the rib being manipulated and the one above.
5. The guiding hand holds the patient's arm.

Procedure

1. The manipulating hand guides the rib into expiration as the patient exhales and resists inspiration as the patient inhales.
2. The guiding hand controls the position of the patient's arm.

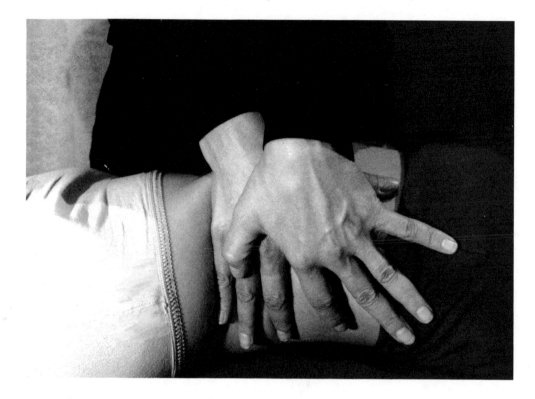

Inspiration Manipulation: First Technique (Fig 11–14)

Purpose

- To increase joint play in the articulations at ribs 5 through 7
- To increase range of motion into pump-handle and bucket-handle inspiration at ribs 5 through 7
- To reduce an expiration positional fault in ribs 5 through 7
- To decrease pain in the thoracic area
- To increase nutrition to articular structures

Positioning

1. The patient is supine.
2. The trunk is in midrange position.
3. The clinician is at the patient's side facing the patient's trunk.
4. The manipulating hand is positioned on the anterolateral surface of the trunk with the volar surface of the index finger between the rib being manipulated and the one below.
5. The guiding hand is positioned over the manipulating hand.

Procedure

1. The manipulating hand guides the rib into inspiration as the patient inhales and resists expiration as the patient exhales.
2. The guiding hand controls the position of the manipulating hand.

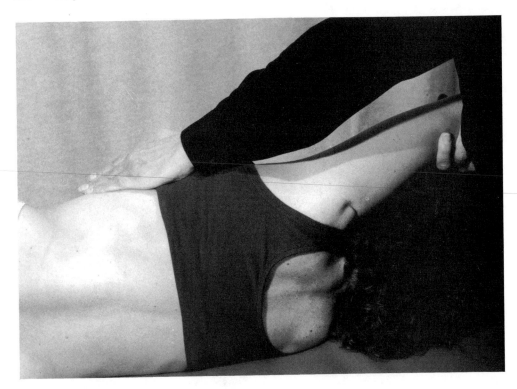

Inspiration Manipulation: Second Technique (Fig 11–15)

Purpose

- To increase joint play in the articulations at ribs 7 through 12
- To increase range of motion into bucket-handle inspiration at ribs 7 through 12
- To reduce an expiration positional fault in ribs 7 through 12
- To decrease pain in the thoracic area
- To increase nutrition to articular structures

Positioning

1. The patient is side-lying with the arm positioned over the head.
2. The trunk is in midrange position.
3. The clinician is at the patient's head, facing the patient's trunk.
4. The manipulating hand is positioned on the lateral surface of the trunk with the ulnar border of the hand between the rib being manipulated and the one below.
5. The guiding hand holds the patient's arm.

Procedure

1. The manipulating hand guides the rib into inspiration as the patient inhales and resists expiration as the patient exhales.
2. The guiding hand controls the position of the patient's arm.

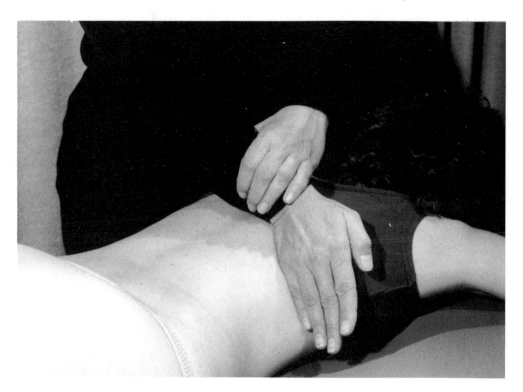

Ventral Glide (Fig 11–16)

Purpose

- To increase joint play in the rib articulations
- To increase range of motion into thoracic rotation to the opposite side as that of the manipulating hand
- To reduce a dorsal positional fault at the ribs
- To decrease pain in the thoracic area
- To increase nutrition to articular structures

Positioning

1. The patient is prone.
2. The trunk is in midrange position.
3. The clinician is at the patient's side facing the patient's trunk.
4. The manipulating hand is positioned with the ulnar border of the hand on the rib being manipulated.
5. The guiding hand is positioned over the manipulating hand.

Procedure

1. The manipulating hand glides the rib ventrally as the patient exhales.
2. The guiding hand controls the position of the manipulating hand.

REFERENCES

1. Grieve GP: *Common Vertebral Joint Problems,* ed 2. New York, Churchill Livingstone, 1988.
2. Saumarez RC: An analysis of possible movements of human upper rib cage. *J Appl Physiol* 1986; 60:678.
3. Veldhuizen AG, Scholten PJM: Kinematics of the scoliotic spine as related to the normal spine. *Spine* 1987; 12:852.
4. White AA, Panjabi MM: Clinical biomechanics of the spine, ed 2. Philadelphia, JB Lippincott Co, 1990.

Figure 12–1

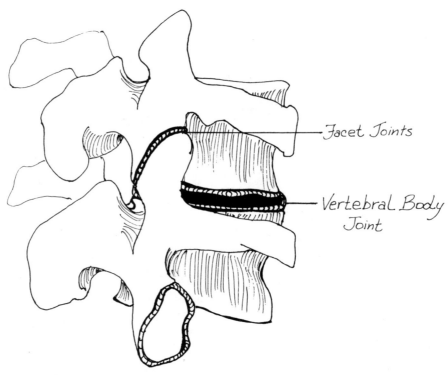

Facet Joints

Vertebral Body
Joint

Lumbar Spine

Chapter 12

Lumbar Spine

FORWARD AND BACKWARD BENDING

Because of the absence of ribs, a greater amount of motion exists in the lumbar spine than in the thoracic spine. As in the thoracic and cervical spines, the degree and direction of movement in the lumbar spine are dictated by the facet joints. The facet joints for the L1 through L4 motion segments are located in the sagittal plane, allowing for a fair amount of forward and backward bending.[7] The L4-5 and L5-S1 facets are aligned more closely with the frontal plane, therefore exhibiting a greater degree of forward and backward bending than in the upper lumbar spine.[7] With forward bending both facets on the most cranial vertebrae glide upward, and with backward bending both facets glide downward.

SIDE BENDING AND ROTATION

Side bending is accompanied by a slight downward glide of the facet joint on the side to which the motion is occurring and a larger upward glide of the contralateral facet joint. Rotation most likely occurs in conjunction with gapping of the facet joint on the side of the rotation and compression of the contralateral facet.[5] Due to facet joint orientation, relatively less side bending and rotation occur at the lower lumbar segments than at the upper lumbar joints.[4,7]

As with the thoracic spine, much controversy exists in the literature as to the existence and nature of coupled motion in the lumbar spine. Coupling most likely does occur with lumbar motion. Side bending and rotation to the opposite side are coupled weakly in the three upper lumbar segments and to the same side in the lowest lumbar segment.[3,4,7] L4-5 is most likely a transitional segment, exhibiting inconsistent behavior.[4] Forward bending and backward bending also most likely are coupled with side bending and rotation; however, the nature of this pattern of coupling has not been delineated clearly because of the complex combination of motions that must be studied.[2,3,6,7] The nature of the relationship between sagittal plane motion and side bending and rotation most likely depends in part on the sagittal position of the spine when motion is initiated, in a manner similar to that hypothesized at the thoracic spine. As with the thoracic spine, many clinicians believe that the pattern of coupled motion in the lumbar spine determines the pattern of limitation. For example, if side bending and rotation to the same side are coupled at the upper lumbar spine, and side bending is hypomobile, then rotation to the same side also will be hypomobile. Restoring motion into side bending will improve motion into rotation. As in the case of the thoracic spine, some clinicians also believe that patterns of restriction occur as a consequence of the position of the patient when injured. This is based on the concept that coupled motion changes based on the sagittal position of the spine.[1] To date there is minimal research to substantiate these claims.

Lumbar Spine

Osteokinematic degrees of freedom:	3 motions:
	  Forward/backward bending
	  Side bending
	  Rotation

Ligaments:	Anterior longitudinal ligament Posterior longitudinal ligament Supraspinous ligament Interspinous ligament Ligamentum flavum Intertransverse ligament
Joint orientation:	Caudal facet of cranial vertebra through L4: ventral, lateral Cranial facet of caudal vertebra through L4: dorsal, medial Caudal facet of L5: Ventral Cranial facet of S1: Dorsal Cranial vertebral body: Caudal Caudal vertebral body: Cranial
Type of joint:	Facets: Synovial Disc: Amphiarthrodial
Articular surface anatomy:	Ovoid, plane Cranial facet: Concave Caudal facet: Convex
Resting position:	Midway between forward bending and backward bending
Close-packed position:	Full backward bending
Capsular pattern of restriction:	Side bending = rotation > back bending

Ventral Glide (Figs 12–2, 12–3)

(It is preferable to perform this technique using the heel of the hand as the mobilizing force. The thumb was used to better visualize the joint.)

Purpose

- To increase joint play in the lumbar spine
- To increase overall range of motion in the lumbar spine
- To decrease pain in the lumbar region
- To increase nutrition to articular structures

Positioning

1. The patient is prone.
2. The lumbar spine is in the resting position.
3. The clinician is standing at the patient's side facing the lumbar spine.
4. The manipulating hand is positioned with the heel of the hand or the thumb over the thumb of the guiding hand.
5. The guiding hand is positioned with the thumb over the spinous process being manipulated.

Procedure

1. The manipulating hand glides the spinous process ventrally.
2. The guiding hand controls the position of the manipulating hand.

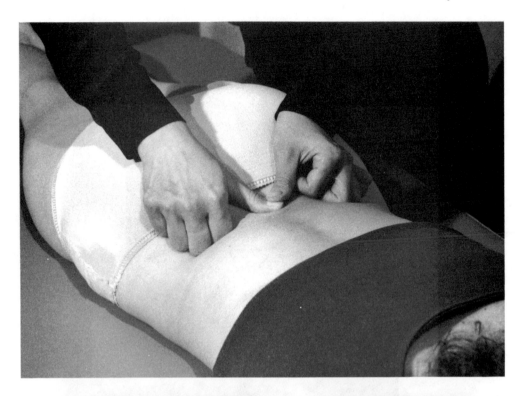

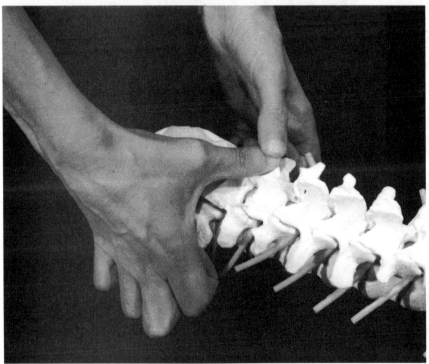

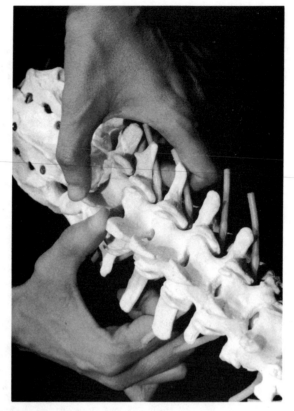

Cranial Glide: First Technique (Fig 12–4)

(It is preferable to perform this technique using the pisiform as the mobilizing force. The thumb was used to better visualize the joint.)

Purpose

- To increase joint play in the lumbar spine
- To increase range of motion into forward bending in the lumbar spine
- To reduce a backward bent positional fault in the lumbar spine
- To decrease pain in the lumbar region
- To increase nutrition to articular structures

Positioning

1. The patient is prone.
2. The lumbar spine is in the resting position.
3. The clinician is standing at the patient's side facing the lumbar spine.
4. The stabilizing hand is positioned with the thumb on the spinous process of the more caudal vertebra.
5. The manipulating hand is positioned with the pisiform or thumb over the most caudal surface of the spinous process of the more cranial vertebra.

Procedure

1. The stabilizing hand holds the vertebra in position.
2. The manipulating hand glides the spinous process cranially and ventrally.

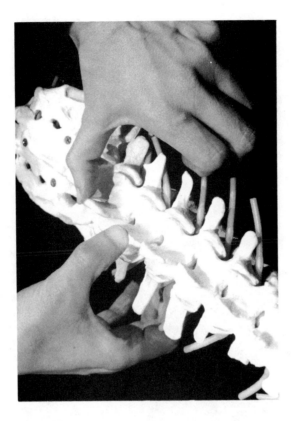

Cranial Glide: Second Technique (Fig 12–5)

(It is preferable to perform this technique using the pisiform as the mobilizing force. The thumb was used to better visualize the joints.)

Purpose

- To increase joint play in the lumbar spine
- To increase range of motion into backward bending in the lumbar spine
- To reduce a forward bent positional fault in the lumbar spine
- To decrease pain in the lumbar region
- To increase nutrition to articular structures

Positioning

1. The patient is prone.
2. The lumbar spine is in the resting position.
3. The clinician is standing at the patient's side facing the lumbar spine.
4. The stabilizing hand is positioned with the thumb on the spinous process of the more cranial vertebra.
5. The manipulating hand is positioned with the pisiform or thumb over the most caudal surface of the spinous process of the more caudal vertebra.

Procedure

1. The stabilizing hand holds the vertebra in position.
2. The manipulating hand glides the spinous process cranially and ventrally.

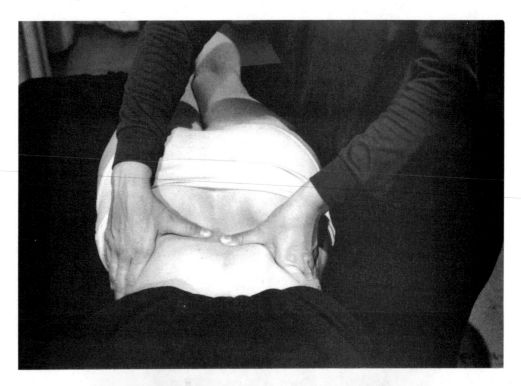

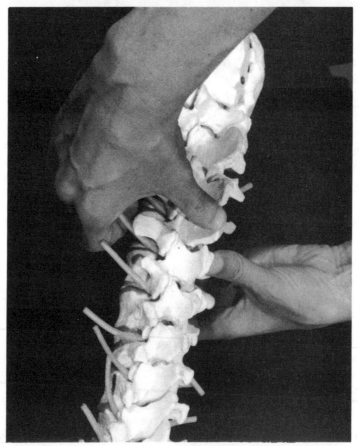

Rotation Manipulation: First Technique (Figs 12–6, 12–7)

Purpose

- To increase joint play in the lumbar spine
- To increase overall range of motion in the lumbar spine
- To increase range of motion into lumbar rotation to the same side as the side of the manipulating hand
- To reduce a lumbar rotational positional fault which is positioned toward the direction opposite the side of the manipulating hand
- To decrease pain in the lumbar region
- To increase nutrition to articular structures

Positioning

1. The patient is prone
2. The lumbar spine is in the resting position.
3. The clinician is standing at the patient's side facing the lumbar spine.
4. The stabilizing hand is positioned with the thumb on the lateral surface of the spinous process of the more caudal vertebra opposite the side to which the vertebra is being manipulated.
5. The manipulating hand is positioned with the thumb on the lateral surface of the spinous process of the more cranial vertebra on the same side as the side to which the vertebra is being manipulated.

Procedure

1. The stabilizing hand holds the more caudal vertebra in position.
2. The manipulating hand glides the more cranial spinous process in a medial direction, thus rotating the vertebra being manipulated on the vertebra below it.

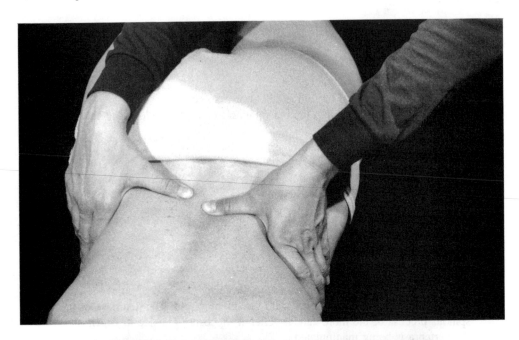

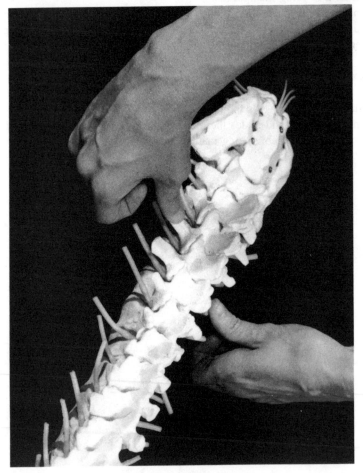

Rotation Manipulation: Second Technique (Figs 12–8, 12–9)

(It is preferable to perform this technique using the pisiform. The thumb was used to better visualize the joint.)

Purpose

- To increase joint play in the lumbar spine
- To increase overall range of motion in the lumbar spine
- To increase range of motion into lumbar rotation opposite the side of the manipulating hand
- To reduce a lumbar rotational positional fault, which is positioned toward the same side as the side of the manipulating hand
- To decrease pain in the lumbar region
- To increase nutrition to articular structures

Positioning

1. The patient is prone.
2. The lumbar spine is in the resting position.
3. The clinician is standing at the patient's side facing the lumbar spine.
4. The stabilizing hand is positioned with the pisiform or thumb on the transverse process of the more caudal vertebra on the same side as the side to which the vertebra is being manipulated.
5. The manipulating hand is positioned with the pisiform or thumb on the transverse process of the more cranial vertebra opposite the side to which the vertebra is being manipulated.

Procedure

1. The stabilizing hand holds the more caudal vertebra in position.
2. The manipulating hand glides the more cranial transverse process in a ventral direction, thus rotating the vertebra being manipulated on the vertebra below it.
3. L5 cannot be treated with this technique, as the iliac crest obscures the transverse processes.

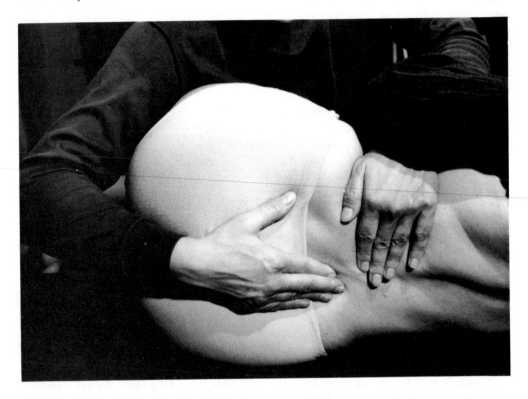

Rotation Manipulation: Third Technique (Fig 12–10)

Purpose

- To increase joint play in the lumbar spine
- To increase overall range of motion in the lumbar spine
- To increase range of motion into lumbar rotation to the same side as the side to which the trunk is turned
- To reduce a lumbar rotational positional fault, which is positioned toward the direction opposite the side to which the trunk is turned
- To release impinged meniscoid tissue
- To reduce a herniated lumbar disc
- To decrease pain in the lumbar region
- To increase nutrition to articular structures

Positioning

1. The patient is lying on his side with his arm resting over the clinician's manipulating arm.
2. The lumbar spine is in the resting position.
3. The clinician is standing facing the patient's side.
4. The clinician locks the the more caudal vertebra by bringing the patient's knees toward his chest to the extent that the motion segment below the one being manipulated is fully flexed, but the motion segment being manipulated has not yet moved.
5. The clinician next locks the more cranial vertebra by rotating the upper trunk away from the treatment table to the extent that the motion segment above the one being

manipulated is fully rotated, but the motion segment being manipulated has not yet moved.

6. The stabilizing hand is positioned with the thumb or index finger on the lateral surface of the spinous process of the more caudal vertebra on the opposite side as the side to which the vertebra is being manipulated.

7. The manipulating hand is positioned with the thumb or index finger on the lateral surface of the spinous process of the more cranial vertebra on the same side as the side to which the vertebra is being manipulated.

Procedure

1. The stabilizing hand holds the more caudal vertebra in position.

2. The manipulating hand glides the more cranial spinous process in a medial direction as the clinician leans on the patient's trunk, thus imparting a rotational force to the vertebra.

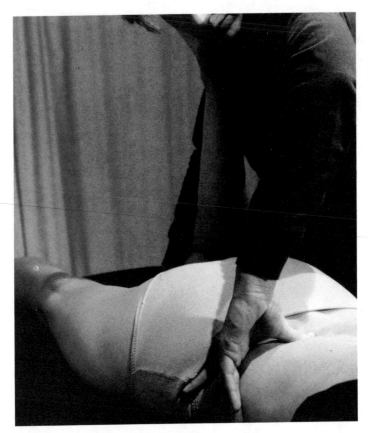

Side Bending Manipulation (Fig 12–11)

Purpose

- To increase joint play in the lumbar spine
- To increase range of motion into lumbar side bending to the same side as the side of the manipulating hand
- To reduce a lumbar side bent positional fault, which is positioned toward the direction opposite the side of the manipulating hand
- To decrease pain in the lumbar region
- To increase nutrition to articular structures

Positioning

1. The patient is prone.
2. The lumbar spine is in the resting position.
3. The clinician is standing facing the patient's side.
4. The stabilizing hand is positioned with the thumb on either side of the lateral surface of the spinous process of the more cranial vertebra.
5. The manipulating hand is positioned on the medial surface of the distal thigh with the clinician's arm and trunk supporting the patient's lower leg.

Procedure

1. The stabilizing hand holds the vertebra in position.
2. The manipulating hand brings the leg into abduction, thus imparting a side-bending force to the more caudal vertebra.

REFERENCE

1. Bourdillon JF, Day EA: *Spinal Manipulation,* ed 4. Norwalk, Conn, Appleton & Lange, 1987.
2. Kulak RF et al: Biomechanical characteristics of vertebral motion segments and intervertebral discs. *Orthop Clin North Am* 1975; 6:121.
3. Panjabi M et al: How does posture affect coupling in the lumbar spine? *Spine* 1989; 14:1002.
4. Pearcy MJ, Tibrewal SB: Axial rotation and lateral bending in the normal lumbar spine measured by three-dimensional radiography. *Spine* 1984; 9:582.
5. Soderberg GL: *Kinesiology.* Baltimore, Williams & Wilkins, 1986.
6. Veldhuizen AG, Scholten PJM: Kinematics of the scoliotic spine as related to the normal spine. *Spine* 1987; 12:852.
7. White AA, Panjabi MM: *Clinical Biomechanics of the Spine.* ed 2. Philadelphia, JB Lippincott Co, 1990.

Figure **13−1**

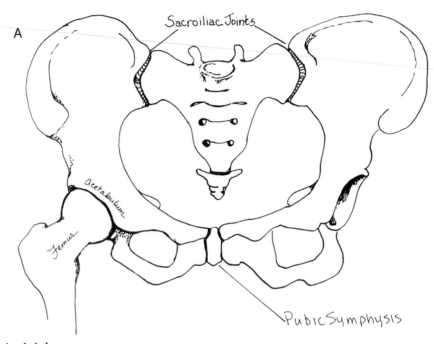

A

Sacroiliac Joints

Acetabulum

Femur

Pubic Symphysis

Pelvic Joints

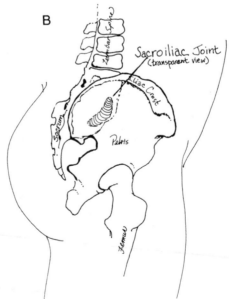

B

Lumbar Spine

Sacroiliac Joint
(transparent view)

Iliac Crest

Sacrum

Pelvis

Femur

Sacroiliac Joint

Pelvic Joints

FORWARD AND BACKWARD TORSION

The pelvic ring consists of three joints: two sacroiliac joints and one pubic joint. Movement at these joints is minimal and does not depend on muscular control.[2] Motion at the sacroiliac joints is greater in women,[1] and decreases with age in both sexes[1, 2, 8] because of progressive roughening of the iliac articular surfaces.[10] Rotation is the predominant motion at the ilia and is characterized by forward and backward movement of the iliac crests. Forward torsion of the ilia is accompanied by counternutation, or extension of the sacrum, and backward torsion of the ilia is accompanied by nutation, or flexion of the sacrum.[7] These motions are accompanied by a translation of some type, most likely in the frontal or transverse plane, or both.[1, 4, 9] Motion at the sacroiliac joint often is identified by the type of movement at the adjacent joints responsible for producing the sacroiliac joint motion. Lumbar movement produces motion of the sacrum on the ilium, or sacroiliac joint motion, and leg movement produces motion of the ilia on the sacrum, or iliosacral movement.[1] Symmetric trunk or leg motion appears to be accompanied by symmetric ilial motion and sacral nutation or counternutation, whereas asymmetric trunk or leg motion is accompanied by asymmetric ilial motion and some combination of side bending, rotation, and forward/backward bending of the sacrum.[1] Any movement at the sacroiliac joints produces motion at the symphysis pubis. This most often is described as a gliding movement in a cranial/caudal direction,[6] although pivoting of the two articular surfaces also has been demonstrated.[5]

Sacroiliac joint disease commonly is due to hypermobility, which often results in a positional fault. When evaluating the sacroiliac joint for dysfunction, it therefore is important to check for both mobility and positional patterns. The most common positional fault occurs when one ilium rotates either in a forward or backward direction on the sacrum, and may occur in conjunction with a sacral positional fault and/or a positional fault at the symphysis pubis. In many cases, treating the ilial positional fault also will correct any sacral and pelvic positional faults that may be present. Many other positional faults of both the sacrum and the ilia have been described in the literature; however, they are not common sources of dysfunction, and in most cases the corresponding physiologic motion has not been ascertained through research.

Pelvic Joints

Osteokinematic degrees of freedom:	Ilia: 1 motion:
	    Forward/backward torsion
	Sacrum: 3 motions:
	    Nutation/counternutation
	    Side bending
	    Rotation

Ligaments:	Sacroiliac joint:
	    Posterior sacroiliac ligaments
	       (transverse, oblique, longitudinal)
	    Anterior sacroiliac ligament
	    Iliolumbar ligament
	    Sacrospinous ligament
	    Sacrotuberous ligament
	    Pubis symphysis: Arcuate ligament

Joint orientation:	Sacrum: Dorsal, cranial Ilia: Ventral, caudal Pubic bones: Medial
Type of joint:	Sacroiliac joint: Part synovial, part syndesmosis Pubis symphysis: Syndesmosis
Articular surface anatomy:	Ovoid Sacrum: Concave Ilia: Convex Pubic bones: Biconcave
Resting position:	Not described
Close-packed position:	Not described
Capsular pattern of restriction:	For both joints, pain when the joints are stressed

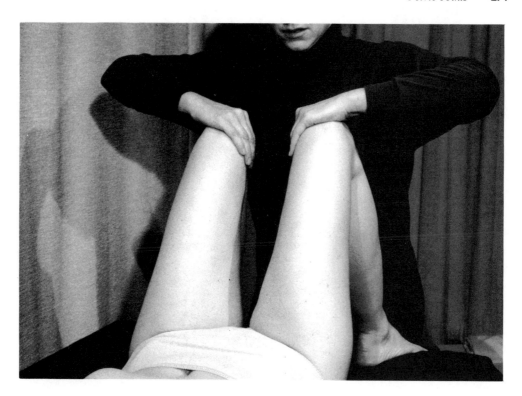

Distraction of Pubis Symphysis: Muscle Energy (Fig 13–2)

Purpose

• To reduce a positional fault at the pubis symphysis

Positioning

1. The patient is supine with the knees bent, feet flat on the treatment table, and hips slightly abducted.
2. The pelvis is in a neutral position.
3. The clinician is at the patient's side facing the pelvis.
4. Both hands are positioned such that each hand is on the medial aspect of each of the patient's knees.

Procedure

1. The clinician instructs the patient to perform an isometric contraction of the adductors by asking the patient to resist a force provided by the clinician into hip abduction, thus distracting the pubis symphysis joint surfaces away from one another as the adductors contract and pull on their attachments to the pubic rami.
2. The clinician then brings the hips into more abduction until an increase in resistance is met.
3. This procedure can be repeated several times.

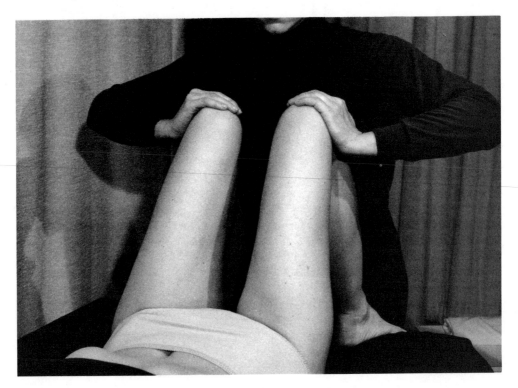

Distraction of Sacroiliac Joint: Muscle Energy (Fig 13–3)

Purpose

- To reduce a positional fault at the sacroiliac joint

Positioning

1. The patient is supine with the knees bent, feet flat on the treatment table, and hips slightly abducted.
2. The pelvis is in a neutral position.
3. The clinician is at the patient's side facing the pelvis.
4. Both hands are positioned such that each hand is on the lateral aspect of each of the patient's knees.

Procedure

1. The clinician instructs the patient to perform an isometric contraction of the abductors by asking the patient to resist a force provided by the clinician into hip adduction, thus distracting the iliac joint surfaces away from the sacrum as the abductors contract and pull on their attachments to the iliac crest.
2. The clinician then brings the hips into more adduction.
3. This procedure can be repeated several times.

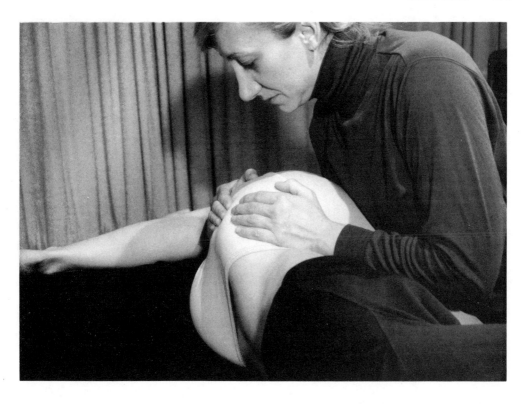

Backward Torsion Manipulation: First Technique (Fig 13–4)

Purpose

- To increase joint play in the sacroiliac joint
- To increase range of motion into sacroiliac backward torsion
- To reduce a forward torsion positional fault of the ilium on the sacrum

Positioning

1. The patient is lying on the unaffected side, with the side to be manipulated positioned with the hip flexed to the end of the available range and the unaffected side positioned with the hip extended and the knee flexed.
2. The sacroiliac joint is approximating the restricted range into backward torsion.
3. The clinician is at the patient's side facing the pelvis.
4. The manipulating hand is on the patient's ischium.
5. The guiding hand is on the patient's anterior superior iliac spine and the ventral surface of the iliac crest.

Procedure

1. The manipulating hand glides the ischium ventrally, thus rotating the pelvis into backward torsion.
2. The guiding hand glides the anterior superior iliac spine and the ventral surface of the iliac crest in a dorsal and cranial direction.

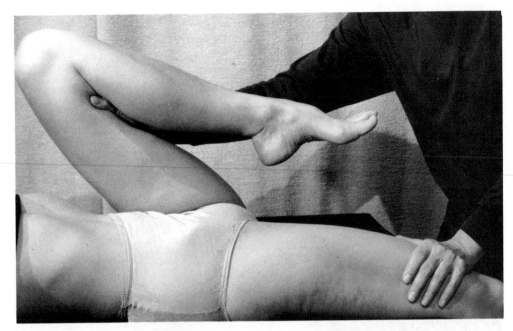

Backward Torsion Manipulation: Second Technique, Muscle Energy (Fig 13–5)

Purpose

- To increase joint play in the sacroiliac joint
- To increase range of motion into sacroiliac backward torsion
- To reduce a forward torsion positional fault of the ilium on the sacrum

Positioning

1. The patient is supine, with the side to be manipulated positioned with the hip flexed to the end of the available range and the unaffected side positioned with the hip extended and knee flexed off the end of the treatment table.
2. The sacroiliac joint is approximating the restricted range into backward torsion.
3. The clinician is at the patient's knee facing the pelvis.
4. The stabilizing hand is positioned on the ventral surface of the distal thigh on the unaffected side.
5. The manipulating hand is positioned on the dorsal surface of the distal thigh on the affected side with the clinician's trunk reinforcing the hand position.

Procedure

1. The clinician instructs the patient to perform an isometric contraction of the gluteus maximus by asking the patient to resist a force provided by the clinician into hip flexion, thus gliding the pelvis into backward torsion as the gluteus maximus contracts and pulls on its attachment to the dorsal surface of the ilium.
2. The clinician next brings the hip into more flexion until an increase in resistance is met.
3. This procedure can be repeated several times.
4. This technique can be combined with the first backward torsion technique.
5. The patient can be taught to perform this technique as part of a home program.

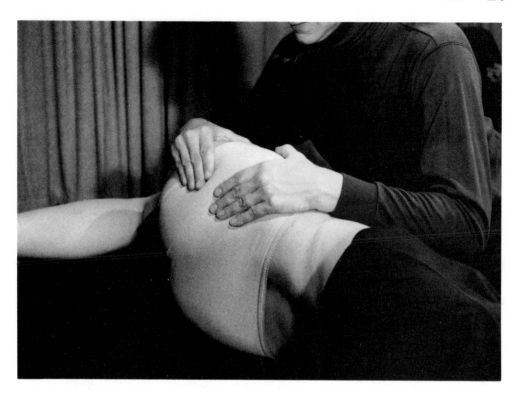

Forward Torsion Manipulation: First Technique (Fig 13-6)

Purpose

- To increase joint play in the sacroiliac joint
- To increase range of motion into sacroiliac forward torsion
- To reduce a backward torsion positional fault of the ilium on the sacrum

Positioning

1. The patient is lying on the unaffected side, with both hips slightly flexed.
2. The sacroiliac joint is approximating the restricted range into forward torsion.
3. The clinician is at the patient's side facing the pelvis.
4. The manipulating hand is over the dorsal surface of the iliac crest.
5. The guiding hand is on the ventral and lateral surface of the pelvis distal to the anterior superior iliac spine.

Procedure

1. The manipulating hand glides the iliac crest ventrally.
2. The guiding hand glides the ventral surface of the pelvis dorsally.

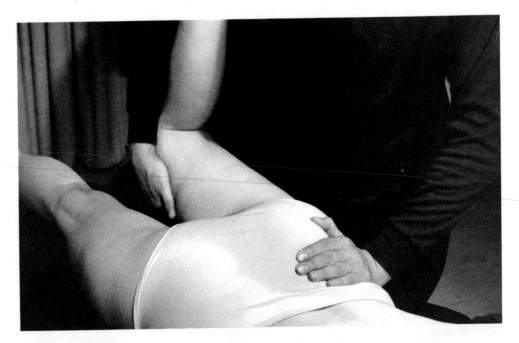

Forward Torsion Manipulation: Second Technique, Muscle Energy (Fig 13–7)

Purpose

- To increase joint play in the sacroiliac joint
- To increase range of motion into sacroiliac forward torsion
- To reduce a backward torsion positional fault of the ilium on the sacrum

Positioning

1. The patient is prone, with the the side to be manipulated positioned with the hip extended to the end of the available range and the knee flexed. The unaffected side can be positioned with the hip flexed off the edge of the treatment table.
2. The sacroiliac joint is approximating the restricted range into forward torsion.
3. The clinician is at the patient's knee facing the pelvis.
4. The manipulating hand is over the dorsal surface of the iliac crest.
5. The guiding hand is on the ventral surface of the distal thigh with the clinician's arm or trunk supporting the patient's lower leg.

Procedure

1. The clinician lifts the thigh off of the treatment table and then instructs the patient to perform an isometric contraction of his rectus femoris by asking the patient to resist a force provided by the clinician into hip extension and knee flexion, thus gliding the pelvis into forward torsion as the rectus femoris contracts and pulls on its attachment to the anterior inferior iliac spine.
2. The clinician next brings the hip into more extension and the knee into more flexion until an increase in resistance is met.
3. This procedure can be repeated several times.
4. This technique can be combined with the first forward torsion technique.

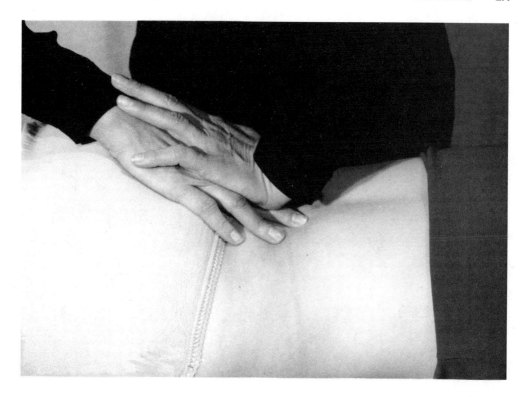

Sacral Nutation Manipulation (Fig 13–8)

Purpose

- To increase joint play in the sacroiliac joint
- To increase range of motion into sacral nutation
- To reduce a sacral counternutation positional fault
- To decrease pain in the sacroiliac joint
- To increase nutrition to articular structures

Positioning

1. The patient is prone.
2. The sacroiliac joint is in a neutral position.
3. The clinician is at the patient's side facing the pelvis.
4. The manipulating hand is positioned over the guiding hand.
5. The guiding hand is positioned over the cranial surface of the sacrum.

Procedure

1. The manipulating hand glides the cranial surface of the sacrum ventrally, thus directing the sacrum into nutation.
2. The guiding hand controls the position of the manipulating hand.

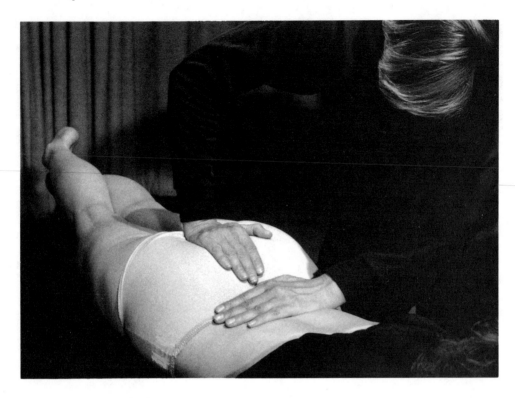

Sacral Counternutation Manipulation (Fig 13–9)

Purpose

- To increase joint play in the sacroiliac joint
- To increase range of motion into sacral counternutation
- To reduce a sacral nutation positional fault
- To decrease pain in the sacroiliac joint
- To increase nutrition to articular structures

Positioning

1. The patient is prone.
2. The sacroiliac joint is in a neutral position.
3. The clinician is at the patient's side facing the pelvis.
4. The stabilizing hand is positioned over the lumbar spine.
5. The manipulating hand is positioned over the caudal surface of the sacrum.

Procedure

1. The stabilizing hand holds the lumbar spine in position.
2. The manipulating hand glides the caudal surface of the sacrum ventrally, thus directing the sacrum into counternutation.

REFERENCES

1. Alderink GJ: The sacroiliac joint: review of anatomy, mechanics, and function. *J Orthop Sports Phys Ther* 1991; 132:71.
2. Bemis T, Daniel M: Validation of the long sitting test on subjects with iliosacral dysfunction. *J Orthop Sports Phys Ther* 1987;8:336.
3. Bowen V, Cassidy JD: Macroscopic and microscopic anatomy of the sacroiliac joint from embryonic life until the eighth decade. *Spine* 1981; 6:620.
4. DonTigny D: Anterior dysfunction of the sacroiliac joint as a major factor in the etiology of idiopathic low back pain syndrome. *Phys Ther* 1990; 70:250.
5. Frigerio NA, Stowe R, Howe JW: Movement of the sacroiliac joint. *Clin Orthop* 1974; 100:370.
6. Grieve GP: *Common Vertebral Joint Problems*. ed 2. New York, Churchill Livingstone, 1988.
7. McGregor M, Cassidy D: Post-surgical sacroiliac joint syndrome. *J Manipulative Physiol Ther* 1983; 6:1.
8. Mierau DR et al: Sacroiliac joint dysfunction and low back pain in school aged children. *J Manipulative Physiol Ther* 1984; 7:81.

Index